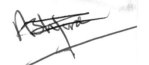
MRCP 1
POCKET BOOK
1

Cardiology, Haematology
and Respiratory Medicine

Second Edition

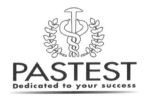

PASTEST
Dedicated to your success

MRCP 1
POCKET BOOK
1

Cardiology, Haematology
and Respiratory Medicine
Second Edition

Paul Kalra MA MRCP
John Paisey BM MRCP
Mary Frances McMullin MD FRCP (Edin) FRCPath FRCPI
Keith Patterson FRCP FRCPath
Howard Branley MB ChB MSc MRCP

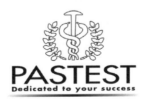

PASTEST
Dedicated to your success

© 2002 PASTEST LTD
Egerton Court, Parkgate Estate,
Knutsford, Cheshire, WA16 8DX

First edition 2002
Reprinted 2002, 2003
Second edition 2004

ISBN: 1 901198 84 7

A catalogue record for this book is available from the British Library.

The information contained within this book was obtained by the author from reliable sources. However, while every effort has been made to ensure its accuracy, no responsibilty for loss, damage or injury occasioned to any person acting or refraining from action as a result of information contained herein can be accepted by the publishers or author.

PasTest Revision Books and Intensive Courses

PasTest has been established in the field of postgraduate medical education since 1972, providing revision books and intensive study courses for doctors preparing for their professional examinations. Books and courses are available for the following specialties:

MRCP Part 1 and Part 2, MRCPCH Part 1 and Part 2, MRCS, MRCOG, MRCGP, DRCOG, MRCPsych, DCH, FRCA and PLAB.

For further details contact:

PasTest, Freepost, Knutsford, Cheshire WA16 7BR
Tel: 01565 752000   Fax: 01565 650264
E-mail: enquiries@pastest.co.uk
Web site: www.pastest.co.uk

Typeset by Breeze Limited, Manchester
Printed and bound by MPG Books Ltd, Bodmin, Cornwall

CONTENTS

INTRODUCTION

PasTest's MRCP Part 1 Pocket Books are designed to help the busy examination candidate to make the most of every opportunity to revise. With this little book in your pocket, it is the work of a moment to open it, choose a question, decide upon your answers and then check the answer. Revising 'on the run' in this manner is both reassuring (if your answer is correct) and stimulating (if you find any gaps in your knowledge).

The MRCP Part 1 examination consists of two papers, each lasting three hours. Both papers contain 100 'Best of Five' questions (one answer is chosen from five options). Questions in each specialty are randomised across both papers. *No marks are deducted for a wrong answer.*

One-best-answer/'Best of Five' MCQs
An important characteristic of one-best-answer MCQs is that they can be designed to test application of knowledge and clinical problem-solving rather than just the recall of facts. This should change (for the better) the ways in which candidates prepare for MRCP Part 1.

Each one-best MCQ has a question stem, which usually contains clinical information, followed by five branches. All five branches are typically homologous (eg all diagnoses, all laboratory investigations, all antibiotics etc) and should be set out in a logical order (eg alphabetical). Candidates are asked to select the ONE branch that is the best answer to the question. A response is not required to the other four branches. The answer sheet is, therefore, slightly different from that used for true/false MCQs.

A good strategy that can be used with many well-written one-best MCQs is to try to reach the correct answer without first scrutinising the five options. If you can then find the answer you have reached in the option list, then you are probably correct.

One-best-answer MCQs are quicker to answer than multiple true/false MCQs because only one response is needed for each question. Even though the question stem for one-best-answer MCQs is usually longer than for true/false questions, and therefore takes a little longer to read carefully, it is reasonable to set more one-best than true/false MCQs for the same exam duration – in this instance 60 true/false and 100 one-best are used in exams of 2 hours' duration.

Application of Knowledge and Clinical Problem-Solving
Unlike true/false MCQs, which test mainly the recall of knowledge, one-best-answer questions test application and problem-solving. This makes them more effective test items and is one of the reasons why testing time can be reduced. In order to answer these questions correctly, it is necessary to apply basic knowledge – not just the ability

to remember it. Furthermore, candidates who cannot reach the correct answer by applying their knowledge are much less likely to be able to choose the right answer by guessing than they were with true/false MCQs. This gives a big advantage to the best candidates, who have good knowledge and can apply it in clinical situations.

Books like the ones in this series, which consist of 'Best of Five' questions in subject categories, can help you to focus on specific topics and to isolate your weaknesses. You should plan a revision timetable to help you spread your time evenly over the range of subjects likely to appear in the examination. PasTest's *Essential Revision Notes for MRCP* by P Kalra will provide you with essential notes on all aspects of the syllabus.

CONTRIBUTORS

SECOND EDITION

Cardiology
Paul Kalra MA MRCP, Consultant Cardiologist, Portsmouth Hospitals NHS Trust.
John Paisey BM MRCP, SpR and Research Fellow, Wessex Cardiothoracic Unit, Southampton General Hospital, Southampton.

Haematology
Keith Patterson FRCP FRCPath, Consultant Haematologist, University College, London Hospital, London.
Mary Frances McMullin MD FRCP (Edin) FRCPath FRCPI, PGCHET, Reader, Consultant Haematologist, Department of Haematology, Queen's University, Belfast City Hospital, Belfast.

Respiratory Medicine
Howard Branley MB ChB MSc MRCP, Raynaud's and Scleroderma Association Research Fellow, National Heart and Lung Institute, Royal Brompton and the Hammersmith Hospitals, London.

FIRST EDITION

Cardiology
Paul Kalra MRCP, Cardiology Research Fellow, Department of Clinical Cardiology, National Heart & Lung Institute, London.
Jeremy Dwight MD MRCP, Consultant Cardiologist, Southmead Hospital, Bristol.

Haematology
Mary Frances McMullin MD FRCP (Edin) FRCPath FRCPI, Senior Lecturer, Consultant Haematologist, Belfast City Hospital, Belfast.
Keith Patterson FRCP FRCPath, Consultant Haematologist, University College, London Hospital, London.

Respiratory Medicine
Howard Branley MB ChB MSc MRCP, Raynaud's and Scleroderma Association Research Fellow, National Heart and Lung Institute, Royal Brompton and the Hammersmith Hospitals, London.
George Ng Wan Kwong MRCP, Consultant Chest Physician, Stepping Hill Hospital, Manchester.

CARDIOLOGY

Best of Five

Questions

CARDIOLOGY: 'BEST OF FIVE' QUESTIONS

For each of the questions select the ONE most appropriate answer from the options provided.

1.1 On clinical examination of the cardiovascular system during inspiration which one of the following findings is consistent with normal physiology?

- [ ] A An increased jugular venous pressure
- [ ] B A diastolic pulmonary venous flow murmur
- [ ] C Increased systemic arterial blood pressure
- [ ] D Decreased pulse rate
- [ ] E Increased splitting of the second heart sound

1.2 A 54-year-old man is admitted with chest pain and ST elevation in the inferior limb leads. He is thrombolysed with streptokinase. During the following 12 hours his blood pressure falls to 80/40 mmHg and his urine output tails off. A central venous line and Swan–Ganz catheter are inserted. His CVP is 15 cmH$_2$O and pulmonary capillary wedge pressure is 20 mmHg. Immediate treatment should include which one of the following?

- [ ] A Inotropic support
- [ ] B Intravenous furosemide (frusemide)
- [ ] C Fluid challenge
- [ ] D Repeat thrombolysis
- [ ] E Rescue angioplasty

1.3 In the electromechanical sequence of action potential and contraction in myocardial cells which one of the following statements is correct?

- [ ] A The plateau phase ends as calcium influx begins
- [ ] B Initial depolarisation of cardiac muscle is the result of a calcium influx
- [ ] C Repolarisation of cardiac muscle is the result of calcium efflux
- [ ] D Calcium ions are required for electromechanical coupling of the cardiac myosite
- [ ] E The energy for contraction of the cardiac myosite is provided by calcium ions

1.4   **On examination of the jugular venous pressure, cannon waves are noted in a patient. These may be due to which one of the following?**

☐ A   The patient not lying at 45°

☐ B   Atrial fibrillation

☐ C   Tricuspid regurgitation

☐ D   VVI pacing

☐ E   Constrictive cardiomyopathy

1.5   **A patient with known stable angina develops chest pain while walking. He stops and takes a dose of GTN spray. The antianginal effect experienced is mainly due to which one of the following?**

☐ A   Reduced platelet adhesion and aggregation

☐ B   Relative bradycardia induction

☐ C   Vasodilatation in response to acetylcholine

☐ D   Peripheral vasoconstriction

☐ E   Plaque stabilisation

1.6   **The clinical sign pulsus paradoxus is observed in which one of the following?**

☐ A   Severe asthma attack treated with positive pressure ventilation

☐ B   Aortic stenosis

☐ C   Aortic dissection causing aortic regurgitation and cardiac tamponade

☐ D   Massive pulmonary embolism

☐ E   Advanced congestive cardiac failure

1.7   **A 35-year-old patient recently arrived from the Indian subcontinent presents with shortness of breath on exertion. A diagnosis of rheumatic mitral stenosis is made. Which one of the following statements is correct regarding mitral stenosis?**

☐ A   The later the opening snap the more severe the stenosis

☐ B   It is approximately equally common in men and women

☐ C   A loud first heart sound suggests a rigid or calcified valve

☐ D   Pre-systolic accentuation of the diastolic murmur occurs if the patient is in sinus rhythm

☐ E   The Graham Steell murmur is due to associated aortic incompetence

1.8   A patient is investigated for a deranged lipid profile. If one of the following conditions is found to be the cause they may be reassured they are at no increased risk of atherosclerosis. Which condition is it?

☐ A   Familial hyperalphalipoproteinaemia

☐ B   Familial mixed hyperlipidaemia

☐ C   Progestogen-containing hormone replacement therapy in post-menopausal women

☐ D   Heterozygous familial hypercholesterolaemia

☐ E   Hypothyroidism

1.9   During the normal cardiac cycle the period of isovolumic left ventricular contraction occurs between the components in which one of the following?

☐ A   The aortic and pulmonary components of the second heart sound

☐ B   The first heart sound and the onset of the carotid upstroke

☐ C   The *a* wave of the jugular venous pulse and the carotid pulse

☐ D   The first and third heart sounds

☐ E   The second and fourth heart sounds

1.10   In secondary prevention of myocardial infarction which one of the following agents has been shown to reduce mortality?

☐ A   Captopril

☐ B   Nifedipine

☐ C   Oral nitrates

☐ D   Verapamil

☐ E   Nicorandil

1.11   Assessment of a typical day-old infant with Fallot's tetralogy may reveal which one of the following?

☐ A   Central cyanosis

☐ B   A widely split second heart sound

☐ C   A chest X-ray showing plethoric lung fields

☐ D   Oligaemic lung fields on chest X-ray

☐ E   Evidence of pulmonary hypertension

1.12 **In which one of the following situations does the exercise tolerance test (ETT) retain most specificity?**

   ☐ A   Hypertension

   ☐ B   Aortic valve disease

   ☐ C   Left bundle branch block

   ☐ D   Hypertrophic cardiomyopathy

   ☐ E   β-Blocker therapy

1.13 **Which is true? Coarctation of the aorta is:**

   ☐ A   Usually acquired but may be congenital

   ☐ B   When congenital, usually associated with brachio-brachial and radio-femoral delay

   ☐ C   A common cause of hypertension in adults

   ☐ D   Associated with an increased incidence of bicuspid aortic valve

   ☐ E   A cause of left-to-right shunting of blood

1.14 **In non-rheumatic atrial fibrillation which one of the following statements is true?**

   ☐ A   The risk of embolic stroke is increased fivefold

   ☐ B   The risk of stroke is greater than in atrial fibrillation due to rheumatic valve disease

   ☐ C   Excess alcohol intake is an unlikely cause

   ☐ D   Cardioversion may be performed without anticoagulation if a transthoracic echocardiogram is normal

   ☐ E   Paroxysmal atrial fibrillation is associated with a lower risk of stroke

1.15 **Regarding Starling's law, which one of the following statements is correct?**

   ☐ A   The force of contraction is inversely proportional to the initial length of the cardiac muscle fibre

   ☐ B   The law is independent of external constraints of extracardiac tissue

   ☐ C   The law means that stroke volume is proportional to left ventricular end-diastolic volume unless the inotropic state of the myocardium or vascular resistance change

   ☐ D   As a consequence of the law, factors which reduce cardiac filling will increase contractility

   ☐ E   The law is dependent on the integrity of the cardiac stretch receptors

1.16 A 63-year-old man presents with palpitations and pre-syncope. A broad-complex tachycardia is recorded on 12-lead ECG. Which one of the following supports a diagnosis of supraventricular tachycardia with aberrant conduction?

- [ ] A Cannon waves are seen in the neck veins
- [ ] B Fusion beats are seen on the electrocardiogram
- [ ] C Atrioventricular dissociation is seen on the electrocardiogram
- [ ] D The patient has a conduction disturbance in their normal rhythm
- [ ] E The tachycardia is of right bundle morphology

1.17 A previously asymptomatic woman becomes breathless during her first pregnancy. Following clinical examination an echo is performed and confirms mitral stenosis. Which one of the following statements is correct?

- [ ] A The lesion has been unmasked by the physiological decrease in cardiac output occurring during pregnancy
- [ ] B A dilated cardiomyopathy of pregnancy is likely to have occurred, unmasking the condition
- [ ] C Most new cardiac murmurs detected in pregnancy are related to stenotic lesions
- [ ] D She should be treated with aggressive diuresis and anticoagulation for the duration of the pregnancy
- [ ] E Pulmonary oedema due to mitral stenosis in pregnancy is usually best treated by valvotomy

1.18 On standing from the supine position compensatory changes in systemic circulation are the result of which one of the following?

- [ ] A Stimulation of the carotid sinus and aortic baroreceptors by a reduced blood pressure
- [ ] B An increase in cerebral Pco_2 and Po_2
- [ ] C Decreased total peripheral vascular resistance
- [ ] D Increased cardiac output
- [ ] E Decreased circulating angiotensin II

1.19   **A 58-year-old man who is taking no medication is referred to Outpatients with palpitations. He has a history of previous anterior myocardial infarction and an echocardiogram reveals moderately impaired left ventricular function. A Holter monitor shows frequent symptomatic episodes of intermittent atrial fibrillation. Which one of the following combinations would be the initial treatment?**

- ☐ A   Digoxin and warfarin
- ☐ B   Amiodarone and aspirin
- ☐ C   Flecainide and warfarin
- ☐ D   Sotalol and aspirin
- ☐ E   Bisoprolol and warfarin

1.20   **A 25-year-old woman presents with a nodal tachycardia and describes terminating the arrhythmia by performing a Valsalva manoeuvre. Which one of the following statements is correct?**

- ☐ A   The manoeuvre is performed by straining to inhale against a closed glottis
- ☐ B   Initially blood pressure decreases slightly, then falls further because venous return is impaired
- ☐ C   A bradycardia is present whilst straining but a tachycardia occurs after release of the manoeuvre
- ☐ D   The heart rate and blood pressure responses are abolished by sympathectomy
- ☐ E   The cardiovascular responses to the manoeuvre may be blunted in diabetes

1.21   **A 65-year-old man presents with shortness of breath on exertion. Examination reveals a displaced apex and a third heart sound. Echocardiography confirms severely impaired left ventricular function. In this patient which one of the following statements is correct?**

- ☐ A   Angiotensin-converting enzyme (ACE) inhibitors and dihydropyridines will reduce mortality by up to 40%
- ☐ B   Digoxin results in symptomatic improvement in patients with a dilated left ventricle and third heart sound only if also in atrial fibrillation
- ☐ C   β-Blockade may result in symptomatic improvement in cases of dilated cardiomyopathy
- ☐ D   A third sound is associated with ventricular ejection
- ☐ E   Treatment with a combination of nitrates and hydralazine is shown to prolong survival in patients on ACE inhibitors and β-blockers

1.22   **A normal infant is born by vaginal delivery. Which one of the following circulatory changes will occur immediately after birth?**

☐ A   Peripheral vascular resistance rises

☐ B   Pulmonary vascular resistance rises

☐ C   Blood flow across the foramen ovale reverses

☐ D   The ductus arteriosus closes

☐ E   Inferior vena caval blood flow exceeds superior vena caval blood flow for the first time

1.23   **A young patient presents with an embolic phenomenon and a myxoma is suspected. Which one of the following is correct regarding atrial myxomas?**

☐ A   They are more common in the right atrium than in the left atrium

☐ B   They do not recur after resection

☐ C   They are distinguished from infective endocarditis by their lack of systemic symptoms

☐ D   They are poorly visualised on echocardiography

☐ E   They usually arise from a pedicle near to the fossa ovalis

1.24   **A 65-year-old lorry driver presents with central crushing chest pain. Which one of the following would suggest a diagnosis of Prinzmetal's or variant angina?**

☐ A   Evidence of proximal coronary artery disease was detected

☐ B   Marked ST elevation with increased R wave amplitude was present during anginal attacks

☐ C   Ventricular dysrhythmias occurred during pain

☐ D   Pain occurred at rest or at night

☐ E   Pain responded well to sublingual nitrates

1.25   **Which one of the following systemic effects are observed in patients with congestive cardiac failure?**

☐ A   Compensatory reduction in basal metabolic rate

☐ B   Inhibition of aldosterone secretion because of sodium retention

☐ C   Polycythaemia

☐ D   Increased circulating renin concentrations

☐ E   Increased responsiveness of the heart to circulating catecholamines

1.26 A 70-year-old man is found to be hypertensive with repeated blood pressure recordings of > 160/95 mmHg. He is already taking a thiazide diuretic. There are no apparent secondary causes of hypertension. He has previously undergone coronary artery bypass grafting. Which one of the following is the most appropriate initial antihypertensive treatment?

- [ ] A α-Blocker
- [ ] B ACE inhibitor
- [ ] C Angiotensin-II receptor blocker
- [ ] D β-Blocker
- [ ] E Calcium-channel antagonist

1.27 A 45-year-old man presents with a protracted episode of central chest pain. He is a current smoker with a strong family history of premature coronary artery disease. His resting ECG is normal. Which one of these investigations would be the most helpful in assisting with planning initial management?

- [ ] A Angiogram
- [ ] B Echocardiogram
- [ ] C Exercise test
- [ ] D Troponin I level
- [ ] E Ventilation/perfusion scan

1.28 A 70-year-old lady presents with severe chest pain and nausea. Examination reveals a pulse rate of 40 bpm, blood pressure 120/60 mmHg and clear lung fields. Her ECG confirms significant inferior ST-segment elevation with complete heart block (CHB). She has received 300 mg of oral aspirin. Which one of the following would be the next therapeutic manoeuvre?

- [ ] A External pacing
- [ ] B Isoprenaline infusion
- [ ] C Thrombolysis with streptokinase
- [ ] D Thrombolysis with tissue plasminogen activator
- [ ] E Temporary pacing-wire insertion

1.29 A 72-year-old man complains of limiting exertional chest tightness. He has clinical evidence of significant aortic stenosis. Transthoracic echocardiography demonstrates a peak aortic valve gradient of 80 mmHg with moderate left ventricular function and probable aortic incompetence. Cardiac catheterisation is performed. What would be the most helpful information to obtain from this investigation?

- [ ] A Aortic valve gradient
- [ ] B Left ventricular function
- [ ] C Presence of co-existing coronary artery disease
- [ ] D Right heart pressures
- [ ] E Severity of co-existing aortic incompetence

1.30 A patient with dilated cardiomyopathy and permanent atrial fibrillation (AF) has a resting heart rate of 110 bpm. Twenty-four-hour taped recordings show even higher uncontrolled rates, particularly associated with exercise. He is already taking 187.5 mg of digoxin and has a normal creatinine. Which one of the following would be the most beneficial treatment?

- [ ] A Addition of β-blocker
- [ ] B Addition of verapamil
- [ ] C AV node ablation and permanent pacemaker insertion
- [ ] D DC cardioversion
- [ ] E Increase digoxin to 250 mg

1.31 A 30-year-old window cleaner has a one-year history of frequent, rapid, irregular palpitations associated with dizziness, but no actual syncope. He drinks approximately 35 units alcohol per week but is on no regular medication. His resting ECG confirms a diagnosis of Wolff–Parkinson–White syndrome (WPW). Which one of the following is the most appropriate treatment?

- [ ] A Amiodarone
- [ ] B Flecainide
- [ ] C Radiofrequency ablation of the accessory pathway
- [ ] D Radiofrequency modification of the AV node
- [ ] E Sotalol

1.32   A 60-year-old lady presents with increasing swelling of the ankles, abdominal distension and dyspnoea. She has a past medical history of pulmonary tuberculosis as a child and a left mastectomy and subsequent radiotherapy five years previously. On examination she is apyrexial, with a sinus tachycardia of 100 bpm and blood pressure of 110/60 mmHg (paradox 8 mmHg). She has significant peripheral oedema and ascites. Her JVP is elevated at   8 cm above the sternal angle and demonstrates a rapid *y* descent. What is the most likely diagnosis?

- [ ]   A   Cardiac tamponade
- [ ]   B   Constrictive pericarditis
- [ ]   C   Intra-abdominal neoplasm
- [ ]   D   Severe tricuspid incompetence
- [ ]   E   Superior vena cava obstruction

1.33   The following findings are obtained during right and left heart catheterisation in a 50-year-old woman:
Pressures (mmHg): right atrial = mean 9, right ventricle = 35/2, pulmonary artery = 36/14, pulmonary capillary wedge = mean 10, aorta = 120/65.
Saturations (%): superior vena cava = 65, right atrial = 76, right ventricle = 77, pulmonary artery = 75, aorta = 97.
She has no significant past medical history, except recent onset of paroxysmal atrial flutter. What is the most likely diagnosis?

- [ ]   A   ASD – ostium primum
- [ ]   B   ASD – ostium secundum
- [ ]   C   Sinus venosus defect
- [ ]   D   Tricuspid incompetence
- [ ]   E   VSD

1.34 An asymptomatic 45-year-old man is noted to have a systolic murmur. He is in sinus rhythm. Transthoracic echocardiography demonstrates normal left ventricular function and dimensions, together with moderate mitral regurgitation secondary to posterior mitral valve leaflet prolapse. The left atrium is enlarged at 4.5 cm. Which one of the following is the most appropriate course of action?

☐ A Amiodarone to maintain sinus rhythm

☐ B Recommend subacute bacterial endocarditis (SBE) prophylaxis and discharge

☐ C Regular clinical follow-up with repeat echocardiography

☐ D Regular clinical follow-up with repeat echocardiography and anticoagulation with warfarin

☐ E Transoesophageal echo and early referral for mitral valve replacement

1.35 A 45-year-old HGV licence holder is seen in Outpatients six weeks after an uncomplicated inferior myocardial infarction (MI), for which he received streptokinase. His resting ECG shows inferior T-wave inversion. What would be the next investigation/procedure?

☐ A Angiography with percutaneous intervention to the right coronary artery

☐ B Bruce protocol exercise test

☐ C Echocardiogram

☐ D Modified Bruce exercise test

☐ E Thallium scan

1.36 A patient presents with severe interscapular pain. Computed tomography (CT) scan confirms a diagnosis of type B aortic dissection. Clinical examination reveals sinus tachycardia of 100 bpm and blood pressure of 150/84 mmHg (similar in both arms). Which one of the following is the most desired intervention?

☐ A Intravenous β-blocker

☐ B Intravenous GTN

☐ C Oral ACE inhibitor

☐ D Referral for urgent surgery

☐ E Transoesophageal echo

1.37 Post-anterior MI, a 60-year-old man develops cardiogenic shock with a blood pressure of 80/50 mmHg and diminished urine output. A Swan–Ganz catheter is inserted and reveals a pulmonary capillary wedge pressure (PCWP) of 20 mmHg; systemic vascular resistance (SVR) 1580 (normal: 900–1200 dyne.s/cm^5) and cardiac index (CI) of 1.8 (cardiac output/body surface area, normal: 2.8–3.5 l/min/m^2). Which one of the following should be the optimal initial treatment?

☐ A   Dobutamine

☐ B   Dopamine

☐ C   Intravenous GTN

☐ D   Intravenous fluids (gentle)

☐ E   Noradrenaline (norepinephrine)

1.38 A patient has a pulmonary embolus, proved by spiral CT scanning. Twenty-four hours after initiation of low molecular weight heparin (LMWH) therapy he becomes hypotensive, tachycardic and hypoxic, without evidence of acute bleeding. His JVP is elevated at 8 cm above the sternal notch. Which one of the following would be the desired intervention?

☐ A   Change LMWH to intravenous unfractionated heparin

☐ B   Inotropic support

☐ C   Insertion of an inferior vena cava filter

☐ D   Thrombolysis with streptokinase

☐ E   Thrombolysis with tissue plasminogen activator

1.39 Six months after prosthetic mitral valve replacement a patient presents with a two-month history of rigors, anorexia, fatigue and weight loss. The CRP is elevated at 110 mg/l. Transthoracic echo confirms moderate paravalvular regurgitation with vegetation. Which one of the following is the most likely infecting organism?

☐ A   *Escherichia coli*

☐ B   *Staphylococcus aureus*

☐ C   *Staphylococcus epidermidis*

☐ D   *Streptococcus viridans*

☐ E   *Candida albicans*

1.40   A 40-year-old male smoker is found to have a fasting cholesterol of
8.0 mmol/l and triglycerides of 1.8 mmol/l. He is hypertensive with a
strong family history of premature coronary artery disease. Which one of
the following would be the recommended intervention?

☐ A   Atorvastatin

☐ B   Bezafibrate

☐ C   Colestyramine (cholestyramine)

☐ D   Diet

☐ E   Pravastatin

1.41   A patient with a previous history of myocardial infarction presents with a
broad-complex tachycardia. Blood pressure is 110/60 mmHg. Lung fields
are clear. What is the most appropriate initial management therapy?

☐ A   Intravenous digoxin

☐ B   Intravenous lidocaine (lignocaine)

☐ C   Oral amiodarone

☐ D   Overdrive pacing

☐ E   Transoesophageal echo and DC cardioversion if no thrombus

1.42   Which one of the following physiological variables has the greatest
influence towards increasing cardiac output during the latter stages of
strenuous exertion in a healthy adult?

☐ A   Coronary vasodilatation

☐ B   Decrease in systemic vascular resistance

☐ C   Increased alveolar ventilation

☐ D   Increased stroke volume

☐ E   Increased ventricular rate

1.43 **A patient undergoes assessment for suitability for percutaneous trans-septal mitral valvuloplasty for the treatment of rheumatic mitral stenosis. The presence of which one of the following features would most likely preclude this form of intervention?**

☐ A   Atrial fibrillation

☐ B   Coronary artery disease

☐ C   Heavily calcified mitral valve

☐ D   Pulmonary hypertension

☐ E   Spontaneous contrast in the left atrium, seen on transoesophageal echocardiography (TOE)

1.44 **An asymptomatic 30-year-old gym instructor is seen as part of a routine medical examination. An ECG demonstrates left bundle branch block (LBBB). Which one of the following clinical signs is most likely to be present?**

☐ A   Displaced apex beat

☐ B   Fourth heart sound

☐ C   Left ventricular heave

☐ D   Reverse splitting of the second heart sound

☐ E   Third heart sound

1.45 **A 15-year-old girl presents with a short history of fever, malaise and a flitting polyarthritis. Clinical examination reveals a soft apical systolic murmur and pericardial rub. Investigations demonstrate elevated inflammatory markers (CRP and ESR). Which one of the following is the most likely diagnosis?**

☐ A   Acute rheumatic fever

☐ B   Atrial myxoma

☐ C   Kawasaki disease

☐ D   Subacute bacterial endocarditis (SBE)

☐ E   Systemic lupus erythematosus

1.46 **A patient undergoes successful elective DC cardioversion for lone AF. Prior to the cardioversion he is taking warfarin, digoxin and verapamil. Which one of the following drugs is the most important for the patient to be discharged on until outpatient review in six weeks?**

☐ A Amiodarone

☐ B Aspirin

☐ C Clopidogrel

☐ D Digoxin

☐ E Warfarin

1.47 **A 40-year-old man is investigated after having undergone successful community resuscitation following an episode of ventricular fibrillation. Echocardiogram demonstrates no structural abnormalities and coronary arteries are normal at angiography. Which one of the following would be the most appropriate long-term management?**

☐ A Amiodarone

☐ B Automated implantable cardiac defibrillator

☐ C Procainamide

☐ D Sotalol

☐ E VT stimulation study and ablation

1.48 **When contemplating coronary artery bypass grafting, which one of the following is the preferred option for revascularising the left anterior descending artery (LAD)?**

☐ A Direct endarterectomy

☐ B Left internal mammary artery

☐ C Radial artery

☐ D Right internal mammary artery

☐ E Saphenous vein graft

1.49   A 30-year-old man presents with recurrent episodes of chest pain and exertional pre-syncope. There is a family history of sudden death. Resting ECG demonstrates features of left ventricular hypertrophy (LVH) and precordial T-wave inversion. Which one of the following is the most likely diagnosis?

☐   A   Dilated cardiomyopathy

☐   B   Hypertrophic cardiomyopathy

☐   C   Ischaemic heart disease

☐   D   Pulmonary embolic disease

☐   E   Supravalvular aortic stenosis

1.50   An infant with trisomy 21 (Down's syndrome) presents with failure to gain weight and clinical evidence of heart failure. Which one of the following congenital cardiac abnormalities is most likely to account for this?

☐   A   Aortic incompetence

☐   B   Endocardial cushion defect

☐   C   Mitral valve prolapse

☐   D   Pulmonary hypertension

☐   E   Secundum ASD

HAEMATOLOGY

Best of Five

Questions

HAEMATOLOGY: 'BEST OF FIVE' QUESTIONS

For each of the questions select the ONE most appropriate answer from the options provided.

2.1   A 65-year-old man is admitted to hospital as an emergency with a cough, a temperature of 40 °C and confusion. He is found to have complete consolidation of the right lower lobe and *Streptococcus pneumoniae* is grown from blood cultures. His blood count shows WBC 13.6×10^9/l, haemoglobin 14.8 g/dl, platelets 503×10^9/l. Blood film examination shows neutrophilia with left shift, thrombocytosis and Howell–Jolly bodies with occasional spherocytes and target cells. In the past he had a hip replacement for osteoarthritis five years ago, and laparotomy and subtotal gastrectomy for peptic ulceration 30 years ago. Which one of the following statements is most correct?

☐ A   Pneumococcal vaccine should be administered prior to discharge from hospital

☐ B   Essential thrombocythaemia with splenic infarction is the most likely cause of his blood film appearances

☐ C   The neutrophil left shift suggests B_{12} or folic acid deficiency

☐ D   He is likely to have had a splenectomy at the time of laparotomy for peptic ulceration

☐ E   Ceftazidime and gentamicin are the most appropriate antibiotics for the treatment of his pneumonia

2.2   A 70-year-old woman is referred to the Outpatient Clinic for the investigation of macrocytic anaemia: WBC 3.2×10^9/l (neutrophils 1.1, monocytes 1.2), haemoglobin 10.6 g/dl, MCV 105 fl, platelets 43×10^9/l. Blood film examination shows hypogranular neutrophils with pseudo-Pelger forms. Which one of the following investigations would be most likely to confirm the diagnosis?

☐ A B_{12} and folate measurement

☐ B   Reticulocyte count

☐ C   Serum ferritin

☐ D   Bone marrow aspirate

☐ E   Haemoglobinopathy screening

2.3 A 14-year-old girl presents with symptoms of anaemia, nosebleeds and purpura of her feet. On examination there is no enlargement of her liver, spleen or lymph nodes. A blood count shows WBC 2.3 × 10⁹/l, haemoglobin 6.0 g/dl, platelets 9 × 10⁹/l. Bone marrow aspirate is hypercellular, showing 95% blasts, a few of which contain Auer rods. Cytogenetic analysis shows translocation between chromosomes 9 and 21. Which one of the following statements about her treatment is true?

- [ ] A If a matched unrelated donor were found then bone marrow transplant in first remission would be her best treatment option
- [ ] B Induction chemotherapy contains high-dose steroids and vincristine
- [ ] C The morphology and cytogenetics are compatible with acute promyelocytic leukaemia
- [ ] D This cytogenetic abnormality is associated with Philadelphia chromosome
- [ ] E Induction chemotherapy would usually consist of cytosine and an anthracycline

2.4 A 35-year-old woman is admitted to the Emergency Department at 8 am after having an epileptic fit on the station platform. A St John's Ambulance volunteer witnesses this. On examination she is confused, has been incontinent of urine, and has a temperature of 37.5 °C. Her husband is contacted at work who states that she has been suffering from a diarrhoeal illness for the last few days and had gone to bed with a headache the previous evening. She has no previous history of epilepsy and is taking no medications regularly. Blood count shows WBC 12.6 × 10⁹/l, haemoglobin 8.6, g/dl, platelets 23 × 10⁹/l. Blood film examination confirms thrombocytopenia and shows occasional fragmented cells. Reticulocyte count is 4.6%. Biochemical tests show normal electrolytes, a creatinine of 146 μmol/l and urea of 8.8 mmol/l. Liver function tests are normal except a bilirubin of 29 μmol/l and LDH 1300 U/l. Which one of the following statements is least likely to be true?

- [ ] A The clinical and pathological features may all be related to the post-ictal state
- [ ] B Increased levels of high molecular weight von Willebrand's factor may be found in her blood
- [ ] C Enteric infection with *Escherichia coli* may be causally related to her illness
- [ ] D The elevated LDH is likely to be of red cell origin
- [ ] E Coagulation screening tests in this disorder are usually normal

2.5   An 18-year-old woman complains of tiredness. She is a vegetarian and her periods last six days of a 28-day cycle. There is no significant previous medical history, and no abnormal features on examination. Blood count shows WBC 4.1 × 10^9/l, haemoglobin 10.1 g/dl, MCV 63 fl, platelets 492 × 10^9/l. Which one of the following is not in keeping with her clinical and pathological features?

    ☐ A   Low serum ferritin

    ☐ B   Stainable bone marrow iron

    ☐ C   Low transferrin saturation

    ☐ D   High erythrocyte zinc protoporphyrin

    ☐ E   Normal haemoglobin A$_2$ level

2.6   A five-year-old boy of Turkish extraction is referred to the school's medical service because of developmental delay. He is noted to be pale and has a palpable spleen. Blood count shows WBC 5.5 × 10^9/l, haemoglobin 4.3 g/dl, MCV 62 fl, platelets 323 × 10^9/l. Which one of the following is not in keeping with a diagnosis of β-thalassaemia major?

    ☐ A   A haemoglobin F level of 90%

    ☐ B   Nucleated red cells in the peripheral blood

    ☐ C   Normal serum ferritin

    ☐ D   Prognathism

    ☐ E   Diastolic murmur at the cardiac apex

2.7   Which one of the following is true of fresh frozen plasma (FFP)?

    ☐ A   It is the optimal replacement fluid following major burns

    ☐ B   Group AB FFP may be given to recipients of any ABO group

    ☐ C   It is approved for the urgent correction of over-anticoagulation with warfarin

    ☐ D   It contains all coagulation factors, albumin and immunoglobulin

    ☐ E   It takes 20–40 minutes to thaw before administration

2.8   A 55-year-old woman on the Intensive Care Unit following a road traffic
        accident has routine haematology investigations performed. These show
        WBC 12.3 × 10⁹/l, haemoglobin 11.4 g/dl, platelets 304 × 10⁹/l.
        Prothrombin time 14 s (control 13 s), APTT 41 s (control 38 s), thrombin
        time 30 s, (control 12 s.). Which one of the following should be done?

- [ ] A   Administration of 2 units of fresh frozen plasma
- [ ] B   Transfusion of 10 units of cryoprecipitate
- [ ] C   Repeat coagulation screen on fresh sample
- [ ] D   Measurement of fibrin degradation products (FDPs)
- [ ] E   Administration of vitamin K

2.9   A 30-year-old woman develops pleuritic left-sided chest pain one week
        after normal vaginal delivery of a six-pound baby boy. On examination she
        is noted to have a swollen left leg and Doppler ultrasound confirms the
        presence of thrombus in the deep venous system. There is no personal or
        family history of thrombosis. Which one of the following investigations is
        most appropriate?

- [ ] A   Measurement of plasma antithrombin
- [ ] B   Coagulation screen
- [ ] C   Screening for factor V Leiden mutation by APC resistance
- [ ] D   Protein S measurement
- [ ] E   Measurement of coagulation factor IX

2.10   The patient above commenced conventional heparin by intravenous
        infusion at a rate of 1000 units per hour. Six hours after starting the
        infusion her coagulation tests shows: INR 1.2, APTT 68 s (control 38 s).
        Which one of the following actions is most appropriate?

- [ ] A   Stop intravenous heparin and give 30 mg oral warfarin
- [ ] B   Convert to therapeutic dose of once-daily subcutaneous low molecular
           weight heparin
- [ ] C   Increase heparin infusion rate to 1500 units per hour
- [ ] D   Continue heparin infusion at current rate
- [ ] E   Stop all anticoagulant treatment

2.11   A 68-year-old woman visits her GP complaining of chilblains. She is noted to have peripheral cyanosis and some screening investigations, including a blood count, are performed. The blood count shows WBC 8.5 × 10^9/l, haemoglobin 10.3 g/dl, platelets 148 × 10^9/l. Film comment is 'heavy cold agglutinates, sample processed at 37 °C'. Which one of the following is the most likely cause of her haematological abnormalities?

☐ A   B cell chronic lymphocytic leukaemia (CLL)

☐ B   Glandular fever

☐ C   Idiopathic cold haemagglutinin disease

☐ D   *Mycoplasma* chest infection

☐ E   Tertiary syphilis

2.12   A 55-year-old man attends his doctor's surgery complaining of a lump beneath his left jaw. On examination he is found to have a mild generalised lymphadenopathy. His blood count shows WBC 50.5 × 10^9/l, haemoglobin 12.6 g/dl, platelets 183 × 10^9/l. Which one of the following would be most against the diagnosis of chronic lymphocytic leukaemia?

☐ A   Peripheral blood lymphocytes expressing both CD5 and CD19 antigens

☐ B   Reduced levels of IgG and IgA immunoglobulins

☐ C   Positive direct antiglobulin test

☐ D   Presence of smear cells on peripheral blood film

☐ E   Balanced expression of kappa and lambda light chain expression of surface immunoglobulin on blood lymphocytes

2.13   A 14-year-old girl with Down's syndrome and epilepsy has a screening full blood count performed after an increase in the incidence of her fits. This shows WBC 4.3 × 10^9/l, haemoglobin 11.0 g/dl, MCV 103 fl, platelets 165 × 10^9/l. Which one of the following should not be considered as a cause of her macrocytosis?

☐ A   Antiepileptic drugs

☐ B   Subacute hepatitis

☐ C   Folic acid deficiency

☐ D   Multiple myeloma

☐ E   Autoimmune haemolytic anaemia

2.14 **Which one of the following statements about blood coagulation is untrue?**

☐ A   The action of antithrombin on fibrinogen results in the development of a fibrin clot

☐ B   Tissue factor is of prime importance in initiation of the coagulation cascade

☐ C   Antithrombin provides a brake on the coagulation system by inactivating excess thrombin

☐ D   Factor IX deficiency results in a prolongation of the APTT with a normal prothrombin time and thrombin time

☐ E   Factor X deficiency results in a prolonged APTT and prothrombin time, with normal thrombin time

2.15 **The mother of a 12-year-old boy with classic haemophilia requests a consultation because of a persistent haemarthrosis of his right ankle. This joint frequently gives him a problem. He is on a regimen of prophylactic alternate-day factor VIII, given by his mother. On examination he has a hot, tender, swollen left ankle. He is otherwise well and there are no other abnormal features on examination. Which one of the following is the most relevant investigation to perform?**

☐ A   Blood count

☐ B   Factor IX level

☐ C   Factor VIII inhibitor screen

☐ D   Urate level

☐ E   Joint aspiration

2.16   **A 25-year-old patient with Philadelphia-positive acute lymphoblastic leukaemia receives a cyclophosphamide/TBI T-deplete marrow transplant from his HLA-matched sister. Both are CMV-antibody negative. Neutrophil and platelet regeneration occur at 21 and 25 days respectively. He also suffered from mild skin graft-versus-host disease, controlled with topical steroid application in the fourth week after transplant. He continued with oral ciclosporin when discharged home six weeks after transplant, but is re-admitted with a dry cough, hypoxaemia, and a chest X-ray which shows bilateral ground-glass shadowing affecting all areas. Which one of the following manoeuvres would not reduce his chance of developing this pulmonary pathology?**

    ☐   A   Transfusion of CMV-negative blood products

    ☐   B   Use of lung shielding during total body irradiation

    ☐   C   Prophylactic monthly nebulised pentamidine during the post-transplant period

    ☐   D   Prophylactic post-transplant itraconazole during the post-transplant period

    ☐   E   Patient immunisation against influenza A pre-transplant

2.17   **A 30-year-old woman is admitted with a deep venous thrombosis. A blood count demonstrates a pancytopenia with a haemoglobin of 5 g/dl and she receives a 4-unit red cell transfusion. Following this she is noted to have dark urine and no red cells are seen in the urine on microscopy. Direct antiglobulin test is negative and repeat blood grouping confirms her ABO type and no atypical red cell antibodies are discovered. Which one of the following investigations is now most appropriate?**

    ☐   A   Donath–Landsteiner test

    ☐   B   MSU for MC&S

    ☐   C   Ham's acid serum haemolysis test

    ☐   D   Urinary haemosiderin

    ☐   E   Measurement of CD55 and CD59 surface antigen on peripheral blood leukocytes and platelets

2.18 **Which one of the following statements about cryoprecipitate is incorrect?**

- ☐ A It is prepared by thawing fresh frozen plasma
- ☐ B It is rich in fibrinogen
- ☐ C It is free of risk of hepatitis transmission
- ☐ D It may correct the platelet defect found in uraemic patients
- ☐ E It contains factor VIII and von Willebrand's factor

2.19 **A 60-year-old woman with high-grade B cell lymphoma receives treatment with CHOP chemotherapy. Ten days after completion of her first course she is admitted to hospital with bilateral bronchopneumonia, requiring treatment with ventilation on the Intensive Care Unit. Her blood count shows WBC 0.9 × 10⁹/l (neutrophils 0), haemoglobin 10.1 g/dl, platelets 106 × 10⁹/l. Which one of the following statements concerning her treatment with granulocyte colony-stimulating factor (G-CSF) is true?**

- ☐ A Prophylactic G-CSF administration to ameliorate neutropenia during future chemotherapy should be administered before and during the course of chemotherapy
- ☐ B Bone pain is a side-effect of treatment which resolves shortly before granulocyte recovery
- ☐ C Extending the time between courses of chemotherapy to allow haematopoietic recovery is preferable to cytokine stimulation of granulocyte recovery
- ☐ D G-CSF carries no risk of viral transmission
- ☐ E G-CSF stimulates haematopoietic stem cells into granulocyte differentiation

2.20 **A 20-year-old woman being investigated for anaemia has the following blood count: WBC 1.6 × 10⁹/l (neutrophils 0.6), haemogobin 7.0 g/dl, MCV 102 fl, platelets 23 × 10⁹/l. Bone marrow aspirate and trephine biopsy are hypocellular, showing residual lymphocytes and scattered eosinophils only. Which one of the following features in her history is not relevant to her diagnosis?**

- ☐ A Recovery from hepatitis A infection three months previously
- ☐ B Recent febrile illness associated with high titres against parvovirus B19
- ☐ C Positive Ham's acid serum haemolysis test
- ☐ D Estranged husband is on busulfan treatment for chronic myeloid leukaemia
- ☐ E Phenylbutazone treatment for ankylosing spondylitis

2.21   **A patient with a first pulmonary embolus has been on continuous intravenous heparin for five days and has received one dose of 10 mg warfarin 12 hours before blood is drawn for coagulation tests: these show an activated partial thromboplastin time (APTT) ratio of 1.7, and an international normalised ratio (INR) of 1.8. Which one of the following is incorrect?**

     ☐   A   The heparin should be increased

     ☐   B   The INR result shows the effect of over-heparinisation

     ☐   C   The patient is unusually sensitive to the effect of warfarin

     ☐   D   The aimed-for INR range in this patient is 3–4.5

     ☐   E   The INR is the patient's prothrombin time in seconds divided by the normal control time in seconds

2.22   **A 60-year-old Asian woman has a haemoglobin of 6.6 g/dl (MCV 63 fl). Which one of the following is least likely to be causally related to her anaemia?**

     ☐   A   History of pernicious anaemia treated with quarterly B_{12} injections

     ☐   B   Regular ibuprofen ingestion for osteoarthritis

     ☐   C   Vegan diet

     ☐   D   β-Thalassaemia trait

     ☐   E   Elevated TSH and low free thyroxine

2.23   **In a patient with chronic renal failure on replacement erythropoietin (EPO) injections which one of the following is not a recognised unwanted effect of this treatment?**

     ☐   A   Hypertension

     ☐   B   Increased risk of thrombosis

     ☐   C   Pure red cell aplasia

     ☐   D   Anorexia and malaise

     ☐   E   Local pain at injection site

2.24 **A 54-year old man has: WBC 5.4 × 10⁹/l, haemoblobin 10.4 g/dl, platelets 135 × 10⁹/l. Differential white cell count shows neutrophils 87%, lymphocytes 6%, monocytes 3%, metamyelocytes 3%, promyelocytes 1%, and nucleated red cells 3 per 100 white cells. Which one of the following is not an appropriate investigation to elucidate the cause of the abnormal blood picture?**

☐ A   Chest X-ray

☐ B   Haemoglobin electrophoresis

☐ C   Bone marrow aspirate

☐ D   Prostate specific antigen (PSA)

☐ E   Abdominal ultrasound

2.25 **Which one of the following statements regarding human blood groups is true?**

☐ A   Naturally occurring anti-A and anti-B antibodies can be both IgG and IgM

☐ B   A minority of people secrete their ABO antigen in saliva and other body fluids

☐ C   The ABO type of individuals can change during some illnesses, eg acute myeloid leukaemia

☐ D   Group A is the commonest blood group in all races

☐ E   Persons of blood group O are universal donors for fresh frozen plasma

2.26 **A healthy blood donor with a haemoglobin of 14 g/dl is found to have a positive direct antiglobulin (Coombs') test. Which one of the following is not an appropriate investigation?**

☐ A   Reticulocyte count

☐ B   Antinuclear factor

☐ C   Clinical examination for enlarged lymph nodes

☐ D   Drug history

☐ E   Barium enema

2.27 **Eight days after commencing intravenous conventional heparin therapy for a deep venous thrombosis a patient's routine full blood count shows a platelet count of 19 × 10⁹/l. This is confirmed on a fresh sample and the records show a normal platelet count on admission to hospital a week before. Which one of the following actions is most appropriate?**

☐ A   Stop heparin and commence heparinoid

☐ B   Change conventional heparin to low molecular weight heparin

☐ C   Stop heparin and commence warfarin

☐ D   Stop all anticoagulant therapy until the results of anti-PF4-heparin complex ELISA are available

☐ E   Stop all anticoagulants and transfuse platelet concentrate

2.28 **A 60-year-old Bangladeshi vegan man is found to have a macrocytic anaemia with low serum B₁₂ level. Which one of the following statements is true?**

☐ A   Parenteral B₁₂ replacement is required monthly

☐ B   Parenteral B₁₂ replacement is extracted from a meat product

☐ C   Measurement of serum levels after parenteral therapy provides a good guide to the efficacy of treatment

☐ D   Measurement of serum levels after oral therapy provides a good guide to the efficacy of treatment

☐ E   Folic acid should be given concurrently with B₁₂ replacement to prevent neurological damage

2.29 A 30-year-old man, previously well, presents to the Emergency Department with a grand mal fit. On examination his temperature is 37.8 °C and he is post-ictal. He has a petechial rash on his lower limbs. His laboratory investigations are as follows: haemoglobin 12.5 g/dl, WCC 10.0 × 10^9/l with a normal differential, platelets 20 × 10^9/l, reticulocytes 205 × 10^9/l (normal range 50–100), PT 14 s (normal range 12–17), APPT 35 s (normal range 24–38) TT 14 s (normal range 14–22), fibrinogen 4.5 g/l (normal range 2–5) D-dimer 0 mg/ml, urea 20 mmol/l, sodium 142 mmol/l, potassium 4.1 mmol/l, creatinine 234 mmol/l, AST 23 U/l, ALT 40 U/l, ALP 95 U/l, bilirubin 40 μmol/l, LDH 950 U/l. Which one of the following is the most likely diagnosis?

- ☐ A Acute glomerulonephritis
- ☐ B Immune thrombocytopenic purpura
- ☐ C Meningococcal meningitis
- ☐ D Systemic lupus erythematosus
- ☐ E Thrombotic thrombocytopenic purpura

2.30 Mr Smith is undergoing a hip replacement. During surgery he loses approximately 1 litre of blood and transfusion of 2 units of packed cells is commenced towards the end of the operation. The anaesthetist notices that his pulse has risen to 130 bpm and his blood pressure has fallen to 80/40 mmHg. He is noted to have frank haematuria. Which one of the following is the most likely cause of the sudden deterioration?

- ☐ A Major ABO incompatibility
- ☐ B Myocardial infarction
- ☐ C Overwhelming sepsis
- ☐ D Reaction to anaesthetic drug
- ☐ E Undetected blood loss

2.31 A 20-year-old thin woman presents with right-sided abdominal pain. In her family history her mother had a splenectomy for anaemia and her maternal grandmother had gallstones. On examination she is mildly jaundiced, tender in her right hypochondrium and has 1 cm of splenomegaly. Ultrasound shows gallstones and an enlarged spleen. Investigations show: haemoglobin 10.5 g/dl, MCV 102 fl, MCH 31 pg, MCHC 35 g/dl, WCC 10.0 × 10⁹/l with a normal differential, platelets 425 × 10⁹/l, reticulocytes 216 × 10⁹/l (normal range 50–100), urea 5.0 mmol/l, sodium 139 mmol/l , potassium 4.0 mmol/l, creatinine 65 mmol/l, AST 25 U/l, ALT 41 U/l, ALP 90 U/l, bilirubin 35 μmol/l, LDH 850 U/l. Which one of the following is the most likely diagnosis?

- ☐ A Autoimmune haemolytic anaemia
- ☐ B Chronic myeloid leukaemia
- ☐ C Hepatitis B
- ☐ D Hereditary spherocytosis
- ☐ E Systemic lupus erythematosus

2.32 A 25-year-old student about to sit his final undergraduate examinations notices that his vision has deteriorated markedly in his right eye. On presentation at the Emergency Department he is noted to be a pale but fit-looking young man. On examination he is found to have 3 cm of splenomegaly and fundal haemorrhages in both eyes, affecting the macula on the right side. A blood count shows haemoglobin 5.5 g/dl, WCC 195 × 10⁹/l (blasts 5%, promyelocytes 10%, myelocytes 34%, metamyelocytes 15%, neutrophils 33%, eosinophils 2%, basophils 1%), platelets 625 × 10⁹/l. Which one of the following is the most likely diagnosis?

- ☐ A Acute myeloid leukaemia
- ☐ B Chronic myeloid leukaemia
- ☐ C Leukaemoid reaction
- ☐ D Myelofibrosis
- ☐ E Primary thrombocythaemia

2.33   A 65-year-old woman has a six-month history of low back pain. She presents to the Emergency Department with weakness in her legs for four days and failure to pass any urine for 24 hours. On examination she is pale and tender over her lumbar spine. Power is grade 4 in both legs with absent reflexes and down-going plantars. Her bladder is palpable to her umbilicus. Her haemoglobin is 10.5 g/dl, MCV 102 fl, WCC 3.0 × 10^9/l with a normal differential, platelets 120 × 10^9/l, urea 20 mmol/l, sodium 143 mmol/l, potassium 4.9 mmol/l, creatinine 300 mmol/l, AST 15 U/l, ALT 22 U/l, ALP 90 U/l, bilirubin 35 µmol/l, total protein 90 g/l, albumin 25 g/l. X-ray of her lumbar spine shows generalised osteopenia and a lytic lesion is noted in her pelvis. Which one of the following is the most likely diagnosis?

☐ A   Guillain–Barré syndrome

☐ B   Metastatic breast carcinoma

☐ C   Multiple myeloma

☐ D   Non-Hodgkin's lymphoma

☐ E   Thrombotic thrombocytopenic purpura

2.34   A 70-year-old woman is noted by her family to be pale and slightly confused. On examination she is anaemic and slightly jaundiced. Pulse is 80 bpm, JVP not raised with a negative hepatojugular reflux and two heart sounds, with no added sounds. Her respiratory system is normal. Haemoglobin 3.5 g/dl, MCV 120 fl, MCH 34 pg, MCHC 35 g/dl, WCC 3.0 × 10^9/l, platelets 105 × 10^9/l, urea 5.0 mmol/l, sodium 141 mmol/l, potassium 4.5 mmol/l, creatinine 65 µmol/l, AST 35 U/l, ALT 32 U/l,   ALP 50 U/l, bilirubin 35 µmol/l, LDH 850 U/l. Which one of the following would be the most appropriate management of this condition?

☐ A   Vitamin B$_{12}$, folic acid and iron supplements

☐ B   Vitamin B$_{12}$, folic acid and iron supplements and slow transfusion of 1–2 units of packed cells if clinically indicated

☐ C   Intravenous folinic acid

☐ D   Immediate transfusion of 4 units of packed cells

☐ E   Transfusion of 4 units of fresh frozen plasma

2.35   A 20-year-old man of Greek origin presents with a three-day history of pallor and dark urine. He was about to go to Kenya on holiday. In his family history a brother had a similar episode some years ago following a course of septrin. On examination, apart from pallor, there is nothing to find. Results show: haemoglobin 5.5 g/dl, MCV 105 fl, MCH 27 pg, MCHC 36 g/dl, WCC 8.5 × 10^9/l with a normal differential, platelets 425 × 10^9/l, reticulocytes 196 × 10^9/l (normal range 50–100), urea 3.5 mmol/l, sodium 138 mmol/l, potassium 4.0 mmol/l, creatinine 70 μmol/l, AST 31 U/l, ALT 27 U/l, ALP 100 U/l, bilirubin 75 μmol/l, LDH 1250 U/l. His blood film shows blister cells. Which one of the following is the most likely diagnosis?

☐   A   Aplastic anaemia

☐   B   Autoimmune haemolytic anaemia

☐   C   Glucose-6-phosphate dehydrogenase (G6PD) deficiency

☐   D   Hepatitis B

☐   E   Hereditary spherocytosis

2.36   A 30-year-old chronic schizophrenic patient is found in a collapsed state. He is unable to give a history but information states that he is taking clozapine, codeine linctus, diazepam, nitrazepam and paracetamol. On examination his temperature is 39.5 °C, pulse 100 bpm and blood pressure 80/40 mmHg. There was nothing else of note on examination. Results show: haemoglobin 12.5 g/dl, WCC 0.5 × 10^9/l with neutrophils of 0.2 × 10^9/l, platelets 220 × 10^9/l, reticulocytes 64 × 10^9/l (normal range 50–100), prothrombin time 13 s (normal range 12–17), APPT 27 s (normal range 24–38), thrombin time 17 s (normal range 14–22), fibrinogen 3.2 g/l (normal range 2–5). Which one of the following is the most likely cause of his neutropenia?

☐   A   Acute myeloid leukaemia

☐   B   Autoimmune neutropenia

☐   C   Clozapine

☐   D   Nitrazepam

☐   E   Septicaemia

2.37   A 20-year-old man has a bone marrow transplant from his HLA-identical
        28-year-old sister for chronic myeloid leukaemia. On day 14 post-
        transplant he develops a rash on his hands and feet. At this time his
        haemoglobin is 10.5 g/dl, WCC 1.0 × 10⁹/l with neutrophils of 0.5 × 10⁹/l,
        platelets 20 × 10⁹/l. On day 16 he experiences vomiting 10 times/day and
        diarrhoea of 2 l/day. His temperature is constantly 37.8 °C despite broad-
        spectrum antibiotics. His investigations on day 16 are: haemoglobin
        10.0 g/dl, WCC 1.5 × 10⁹/l with neutrophils of 1.0 × 10⁹/l, platelets
        15 × 10⁹/l, urea 10.0 mmol/l, sodium 145 mmol/l, potassium 3.0 mmol/l,
        creatinine 200 μmol/l, AST 53 U/l, ALT 61 U/l, ALP 160 U/l, bilirubin
        40 μmol/l, LDH 655 U/l. Which one of the following is the most likely
        cause of his symptomatology?

☐   A   Graft failure
☐   B   Graft-versus-host disease
☐   C   Relapse of chronic myeloid leukaemia
☐   D   Rotavirus infection
☐   E   Veno-occlusive disease

2.38   A 65-year-old woman, a lifelong blood donor, presents complaining of
        arthralgia and increased skin pigmentation. She is a social drinker and she
        has a family history of cirrhosis. On examination she appears suntanned
        and has 2 cm of hepatomegaly. On investigation: haemoglobin 15.5 g/dl,
        WCC 7.4 × 10⁹/l, platelets 315 × 10⁹/l, urea 8.0 mmol/l, sodium
        140 mmol/l, potassium 3.5 mmol/l, creatinine 110 μmol/l, AST 60 U/l, ALT
        75 U/l, ALP 135 U/l, bilirubin 23 μmol/l, LDH 455 U/l, serum iron
        53 μmol/l (normal range 14–29), TIBC 80 μmol/l (normal range 45–72),
        ferritin 985 μg/l (normal range 15–200). Which one of the following is the
        most likely diagnosis?

☐   A   Acute viral hepatitis
☐   B   Alcoholic cirrhosis
☐   C   Excess iron ingestion
☐   D   Haemochromatosis
☐   E   Wilson's disease

2.39 A 70-year-old man presents with a history of tiredness and increasing shortness of breath. On examination he is clinically anaemic. On investigation his haemoglobin is 8.5 g/dl, MCV 110 fl, MCH 24 pg, MCHC 29 g/dl, WCC 10.4 × 10^9/l, platelets 80 × 10^9/l, normal urea and electrolytes and liver function tests, serum iron 45 μmol/l (normal range 14–29), TIBC 64 μmol/l (normal range 45–72), ferritin 453 μg/l (normal range 15–200). Bone marrow aspirate shows abnormal erythropoiesis and increased iron in the stores and erythroid series. Which one of the following is the most likely diagnosis?

☐ A   Acute myeloid leukaemia

☐ B   Haemochromatosis

☐ C   Multiple myeloma

☐ D   Myelodysplastic syndrome

☐ E   Sideroblastic anaemia

2.40 A 20-year-old African refugee presents with sudden onset of a dense right-sided hemiparesis. He speaks little English but from friends it appears that he has no previous medical history of note but two siblings died in infancy. On examination he has a right hemiparesis and 3 cm splenomegaly. On investigation his haemoglobin is 8.5 g/dl, MCV 102 fl, MCH 33 pg, MCHC 32.5 g/dl, WCC 12.5 × 10^9/l with a neutrophil leukocytosis, platelets 120 × 10^9/l, reticulocytes 221 × 10^9/l (normal range 50–100), urea 3.5 mmol/l, sodium 140 mmol/l, potassium 4.0 mmol/l, creatinine 70 μmol/l, AST 30 U/l, ALT 62 U/l, ALP 52 U/l, bilirubin 55 μmol/l, LDH 1128 U/l. His blood film shows numerous sickled cells. Which one of the following is the most important immediate management of his condition?

☐ A   Immediate exchange transfusion

☐ B   Intravenous antibiotics

☐ C   Pain relief

☐ D   Rehydration

☐ E   Top-up transfusion

2.41   You are called to see a 28-year-old Hong Kong Chinese lady who is
28 weeks pregnant (first pregnancy). She has no previous history of note.
She is now pre-eclamptic and the fetus has been noted on ultrasound to be
hydropic. Results show: haemoglobin 10.5 g/dl, MCV 65 fl, MCH 22 pg,
MCHC 37 g/dl, WCC 11.5 × 10⁹/l, platelets 120 × 10⁹/l, prothrombin
time 12 s (normal range 12–17), APPT 29 s (normal range 24–38),
thrombin time 16 s (normal range 14–22), fibrinogen 3.2 g/l (normal range
2–5), urea 9.5 mmol/l, sodium 137 mmol/l, potassium 4.0 mmol/l,
creatinine 110 μmol/l, AST 53 U/l, ALT 52 U/l, ALP 110 U/l, bilirubin
36 μmol/l, LDH 700 U/l. Which one of following is the most likely cause of
the hydropic fetus?

☐ A   HELLP syndrome

☐ B   Hepatitis C

☐ C   Pre-eclampsia

☐ D   Septicaemia

☐ E   α-Thalassaemia major

2.42   A 20-year-old woman presents with a history of shortness of breath and
tiredness. There is no past medical history of note. On examination she is
clinically anaemic and has bilateral fundal haemorrhages. There is a
petechial rash on her ankles. There is nothing else of note on examination.
Her haemoglobin is 3.5 g/dl, WCC 1.0 × 10⁹/l, neutrophils 0.2 × 10⁹/l,
platelets 10 × 10⁹/l. Coagulation screen, urea and creatinine and liver
function tests are all normal. Which one of the following is the most likely
diagnosis?

☐ A   Acute myeloid leukaemia

☐ B   Aplastic anaemia

☐ C   Megaloblastic anaemia

☐ D   Meningococcal septicaemia

☐ E   Paroxysmal nocturnal haemoglobinuria

2.43   A 65-year-old lady had an aortic valve replacement and coronary artery bypass surgery ten days ago. She has been unwell since and has continued to need ventilation. Her ventilatory requirements increase and she is shown on CT scan to have had a pulmonary embolus despite administration of enoxaparin 40 mg/day subcutaneously. Her haemoglobin 10.5 g/dl, WCC 12.5 × 10⁹/l, neutrophils 10.0 × 10⁹/l, platelets 20 × 10⁹/l. Which one of the following is the most likely cause of her pulmonary embolus?

☐   A   Continued ventilation

☐   B   Factor V Leiden deficiency

☐   C   Heparin-induced thrombocytopenia

☐   D   Insufficient dose of Clexane

☐   E   Immune thrombocytopenic purpura

2.44   You are called to investigate a nine-year-old boy who had excessive bleeding following tonsillectomy necessitating return to theatre on two occasions. He has not had any previous history of surgery. His mother has a history of menorrhagia and a maternal aunt bled excessively following tonsillectomy as a child. Results show: haemoglobin 12.5 g/dl, WCC 8.5 × 10⁹/l, platelets 150 × 10⁹/l, prothrombin time 15 s (normal range 12–17), APPT 45 s (normal range 24–38), thrombin time 17 s (normal range 14–22), fibrinogen 3.8 g/l (normal range 2–5). Which one of the following is the most likely diagnosis?

☐   A   Excessive aspirin ingestion

☐   B   Haemophilia A

☐   C   Haemophilia B

☐   D   Surgical bleeding (silk deficiency)

☐   E   von Willebrand's disease

2.45 A 21-year-old primigravida presents at 31 weeks gestation with severe abdominal pain. An ultrasound shows abruptio placenta. A fetal heartbeat is detected so immediate caesarean section is planned. Pre-operatively her haemoglobin is 5.4 g/dl, WCC 16.3 × 10⁹/l, platelets 28 × 10⁹/l, prothrombin time 22 s (normal range 12–17), APPT 52 s (normal range 24–38), thrombin time 34 s (normal range 14–22), reptilase time 31 s (normal range 15–18) fibrinogen 0.8 g/l (normal range 2–5) FDP 120 μg/ml (normal range < 10). Which one of the following is the most likely cause of her coagulation problem?

- ☐ A   Blood loss
- ☐ B   Disseminated intravascular coagulation
- ☐ C   Over-transfusion with colloid (haemodilution)
- ☐ D   Septicaemia
- ☐ E   von Willebrand's disease

2.46 An eight-year-old boy presents with severe pain in the long bones of both legs. His mother thinks that he has had more colds than his two siblings in the last six months. On examination he is pale, temperature 36.8 °C. He is very tender over his sternum and both tibia. There is nothing else to find on examination. Laboratory tests show: haemoglobin 9.4 g/dl, WCC 2.53 × 10⁹/l, platelets 28 × 10⁹/l, neutrophils 0.5 × 10⁹/l, lymphocytes 1.6 × 10⁹/l, monocytes 0.43 × 10⁹/l with a few abnormal lymphocytes reported as seen on the film, normal coagulation screen, normal electrolytes and liver function tests. Rheumatoid factor was negative. Which one of the following is the most likely diagnosis?

- ☐ A   Acute lymphoblastic leukaemia
- ☐ B   Acute myeloid leukaemia
- ☐ C   Aplastic anaemia
- ☐ D   Juvenile chronic arthritis
- ☐ E   Growing pains

2.47   A 24-year-old man has noted for the last two months that his face is swollen in the morning. He has lost 10 kg in weight over six months. He has no other complaints. On examination his external jugular veins are dilated. His chest X-ray shows a mediastinal mass. Which one of the following is the most likely diagnosis of his superior vena caval obstruction?

☐ A   Adenocarcinoma of the lung

☐ B   Hodgkin's disease

☐ C   Sarcoidosis

☐ D   Seminoma

☐ E   Tuberculosis

2.48   An 80-year-old woman presents with a transient ischaemic attack with five minute loss of power in her right side. She has no previous history of note, has been very well and is not on any medication. On examination, when seen, there are no residual neurological signs. On investigation her haemoglobin is 12.5 g/dl, MCV 94 fl, MCH 29 pg, MCHC 33.5 g/dl, WCC 7.5 $\times$ 10^9/l, platelets 1135 $\times$ 10^9/l, ESR 2 mm in the first hour, coagulation screen normal, ferritin 23 μg/l (normal range 15–200), serum B_{12} 600 pmol/l and serum folate 3.0 μg/l. Which one of the following is the most likely diagnosis?

☐ A   Chronic myeloid leukaemia

☐ B   Iron deficiency anaemia

☐ C   Occult neoplasm

☐ D   Primary thrombocythaemia

☐ E   Urinary tract infection

2.49   A 16-year-old is brought by her mother to see you as her mother is worried about her. Her diet is poor. She is vegetarian but is mainly eating bread and chips. Her periods have been very heavy for the last six months. Apart from pallor there is nothing to find on examination. On investigation her haemoglobin is 6.5 g/dl, MCV 65 fl, MCH 22 pg, MCHC 27.4 g/dl, WCC 6.8 × 10⁹/l, platelets 520 × 10⁹/l, coagulation screen normal, ferritin 8 μg/l. Which one of the following is the most appropriate management of her iron deficiency anaemia?

☐ A   Dietary advice

☐ B   Intravenous iron

☐ C   Oral iron supplements

☐ D   Oral contraceptive pill

☐ E   Transfusion of packed cells

2.50   A 60-year-old woman has a long history of asthma and a skin disorder involving a blistering eruption on her elbows and knees. There is no family history of note. She presents with an exacerbation of her asthma precipitated by a flu-like illness. On examination she is noted to have central cyanosis, pulse 100 bpm in sinus rhythm, jugular venous pressure not raised and two heart sounds with no added sounds. In the respiratory system there is good air entry to all areas with widespread expiratory wheeze. Pulse oximetry gave a reading of 89% on room air but P_{O_2} was 14.5 kPa. Which one of the following is the most likely cause of her cyanosis?

☐ A   Congenital methaemoglobinaemia

☐ B   Congestive cardiac failure

☐ C   Methaemoglobinaemia induced by dapsone

☐ D   *Pneumocystis* infection

☐ E   Respiratory failure

2.51 A 23-year-old woman about to complete her final university examinations, presents with abdominal swelling and on investigation is found to have Budd–Chiari syndrome. Results showed: haemoglobin is 12.5 g/dl, PCV 42%, MCV 70 fl, MCH 24 pg, MCHC 29.5 g/dl, WCC 15.5 × 10⁹/l, platelets 835 × 10⁹/l, coagulation screen normal, protein C 80 U/dl (normal range 70–140), protein S 90 U/dl (normal range 60–140), antithrombin 110 U/dl (normal range 80–120), APC resistance 2.38 (normal range 2.35 +/– 0.17), ferritin 14 μg/l (normal range 15–200). She is given oral iron and three weeks later her blood count is: haemoglobin 17.5 g/dl, PCV 55%, MCV 72 fl, MCH 28 pg, MCHC 30.5 g/dl, WCC 14.5 × 10⁹/l, platelets 721 × 10⁹/l. Which one of the following is the most likely cause for her haematological problem?

- [ ] A Chronic myeloid leukaemia
- [ ] B Factor V Leiden heterozygote
- [ ] C Iron deficiency anaemia
- [ ] D Polycythaemia vera
- [ ] E Primary thrombocythaemia

2.52 A 78-year-old man attends his general practice with a one-week history of cough and sputum. He has no past medical history of note and has not seen his general practitioner for ten years. On examination he has coarse crepitations at his right lung base. The chest X-ray shows an area of consolidation at his right base, haemoglobin is 12.4 g/dl, WCC 65 × 10⁹/l, platelets 123 × 10⁹/l, neutrophils 3.5 × 10⁹/l, lymphocytes 58.4 × 10⁹/l, monocytes 4.1 × 10⁹/l, with smear cells reported as seen on the film. Immunoglobins: IgG 5.5 g/l (normal range 7.0–16.0), IgA 0.7 g/l (normal range 0.8–4.7), IgM 0.4 g/l (normal range 0.5–3.0). Which one of the following is the most likely diagnosis of his haematological problem?

- [ ] A Acute lymphoblastic leukaemia
- [ ] B Chronic lymphocytic leukaemia
- [ ] C Hodgkin's lymphoma
- [ ] D Glandular fever
- [ ] E Non-Hodgkin's lymphoma

2.53   A 30-year-old woman has a flu-like illness. Two weeks later she presents
        with widespread bruising and a very heavy period. On examination she
        appears well but has a widespread petechial rash on both lower limbs and
        nil else of note. On investigation, haemoglobin is 11.4 g/dl,
        WCC 5.6 × 10^9/l, platelets 10 × 10^9/l; coagulation screen, urea,
        electrolytes and liver function tests are all normal. Which one of the
        following is the most likely diagnosis?

☐ A   Acute myeloid leukaemia

☐ B   Aplastic anaemia

☐ C   Immune thrombocytopenic purpura

☐ D   Non-Hodgkin's lymphoma

☐ E   Pernicious anaemia

RESPIRATORY MEDICINE

Best of Five

Questions

RESPIRATORY MEDICINE: 'BEST OF FIVE' QUESTIONS

For each of the questions select the ONE most appropriate answer from the options provided.

3.1 **You are asked to give a lecture to a group of first year medical students about normal lung structure and function. Which one of the following statements is correct?**

☐ A The right lung is smaller than the left

☐ B The lingula is anatomically part of the left lower lobe

☐ C The terminal bronchioles lead into the alveolar ducts

☐ D The alveoli have well-established collateral ventilation

☐ E The glottis narrows during inspiration

3.2 **A 63-year-old woman has had repeated urinary tract infections. She now presents with breathlessness and some pulmonary fibrosis is evident on her chest X-ray. Which one of the following is the most likely antibiotic she has been taking?**

☐ A Amoxicillin

☐ B Ciprofloxacin

☐ C Fucidic acid

☐ D Nitrofurantoin

☐ E Erythromycin

3.3 **A 37-year-old man is HIV-positive. He develops breathlessness associated with bilateral shadowing on his chest X-ray. You think he may have *Pneumocystis carinii* pneumonia (PCP). Which one of the following statements is correct?**

☐ A First-line treatment should be with intravenous co-triamterzide

☐ B Diagnosis is by auramine O stain on a bronchoalveolar lavage specimen

☐ C Severe hypoxaemia is uncommon

☐ D This infection is common in HIV-positive Africans with AIDS

☐ E Overall mortality is approximately 10%

3.4   **A physiotherapist on your ward thinks that a patient has an abnormal chest X-ray. You look at the X-ray but which one of the following would you tell the physiotherapist is a normal appearance?**

☐   A   The left dome of the diaphragm is usually higher than the right

☐   B   The hilar shadows are principally composed of lymphoid tissue

☐   C   The left hilum is higher than the right

☐   D   Loss of clarity of the left heart border suggests pathology in the lower lobe

☐   E   The lower trachea is deviated to the right

3.5   **A 25-year-old man consults you with a rash he thinks is chickenpox. Whilst taking a history you discover that he did not have chickenpox as a child and that he is slightly breathless at rest. He thinks he may have chickenpox pneumonia and he has a list of questions regarding this problem and his subsequent management. Which one of the following statements regarding chickenpox pneumonia is correct?**

☐   A   It is commoner in children

☐   B   Patients are still infectious once the rash has appeared

☐   C   It causes upper zone fibrosis on chest X-ray

☐   D   It should be treated with ganciclovir

☐   E   Secondary infection with *Staphylococcus aureus* and *Streptococcus pneumoniae* is common

3.6   **You are comparing pulmonary blood flow in patients with breathlessness to a cohort of normal healthy non-breathless subjects to see if there is a difference. Which one of the following statements regarding pulmonary blood flow in normal subjects is correct?**

☐   A   Pulmonary blood flow is greatest at the lung apices

☐   B   The carotid sinus is a chemoreceptor, monitoring arterial Po_2 and Pco_2

☐   C   Respiration is stimulated when arterial Po_2 falls below about 85 mmHg (11.3 kPa)

☐   D   Mean pulmonary artery pressure is about 30 mmHg (4 kPa)

☐   E   The total resistance in the pulmonary circulation is about 10% of that in the systemic circulation

3.7　　Your surgical colleagues ask for advice about a 62-year-old patient they have who feels weak and is breathless. He is due for an elective repair of an inguinal hernia. They have a lung function request form but are not sure which boxes to tick. Which one of the following pieces of advice you could give them is correct?

- [ ] A　Total lung capacity (TLC) is the volume of gas in the lungs during normal inspiration
- [ ] B　Peak flow is useful in monitoring respiratory muscle weakness in Guillain–Barré syndrome
- [ ] C　A decreased FEV_1/FVC ratio is commonly seen in bronchiectasis
- [ ] D　An increased FEV_1/FVC ratio is commonly seen in bronchiectasis
- [ ] E　Functional residual capacity may be measured directly by spirometry

3.8　　A 59-year-old man with a 30 pack/year smoking history comes to your clinic with breathlessness. You request measurement of his static lung volumes as part of your respiratory work-up. Which one of the following statements regarding static lung volumes is correct?

- [ ] A　May be underestimated using body box plethysmography
- [ ] B　Are decreased in asthma
- [ ] C　Ratio of residual volume/total lung capacity can be increased in chronic obstructive pulmonary disease (COPD)
- [ ] D　When measured by helium dilution technique can overestimate the size of bullae
- [ ] E　May be increased in cryptogenic fibrosing alveolitis

3.9　　A 39-year-old woman with asthma has a strongly positive skin-prick test to *Aspergillus fumigatus*. You think that she might have allergic bronchopulmonary aspergillosis. Which one of the following would best help you to confirm your suspicion?

- [ ] A　Presence of distal bronchiectasis on CT scan
- [ ] B　Following treatment with oral itraconazole, *Aspergillus*-specific IgE decreases
- [ ] C　Absence of peripheral eosinophilia
- [ ] D　Precipitating antibodies to *Aspergillus fumigatus* antigen
- [ ] E　Positive RAST to *Aspergillus fumigatus*

3.10 **A 32-year-old man with cough and breathlessness is found to have an elevated gas transfer factor on pulmonary function testing. There is a family history of cough and breathlessness. What is the most likely diagnosis?**

☐ A   Pulmonary embolus

☐ B   Asthma

☐ C   Anaemia of chronic disease

☐ D   Emphysema due to α_1-antitrypsin deficiency

☐ E   Extrinsic allergic alveolitis

3.11 **A local GP telephones you for advice for one of his female patients who is being treated for pulmonary tuberculosis. He asks you about how the drugs work and what adverse drug reactions he should be on the lookout for. Which of the following pieces of advice is correct?**

☐ A   Pyridoxine is given to prevent pyrazinamide-related neuropathy

☐ B   Anticonvulsant therapy should be reduced accordingly

☐ C   Ethambutol may cause a maculopathy

☐ D   Rifampicin is contraindicated in renal failure

☐ E   Isoniazid is predominantly bactericidal in action

3.12 **You are referred a patient with breathlessness who has previously had a laryngeal carcinoma resected. The ENT surgeon can find no sign of recurrence but can hear some mild inspiratory stridor. Which of the following tests will best help you to decide if there is any element of upper airways obstruction?**

☐ A   Peak expiratory flow rate (PEFR)

☐ B   Ratio of forced expiratory volume in first second (FEV_1) to forced vital capacity (FVC)

☐ C   Flow/volume loop

☐ D   Gas transfer factor

☐ E   Total lung capacity (TLC)

3.13 **A 40-year-old man attends the Respiratory Clinic following a chest X-ray that shows pulmonary shadowing. His blood tests reveal the presence of an eosinophilia. Which one of the following is the least likely diagnosis?**

☐ A Extrinsic allergic alveolitis

☐ B *Ascaris lumbricoides*

☐ C Aspirin

☐ D *Aspergillus fumigatus*

☐ E Polyarteritis nodosa

3.14 **A 74-year-old man with a 60 pack/year smoking history is brought to the Emergency Department with acute breathlessness. The SHO says that arterial blood gases reveal that the patient has a metabolic acidosis. Which one of the following statements concerning metabolic acidosis is correct?**

☐ A Arterial P_{CO_2} is typically normal/high

☐ B Plasma bicarbonate is normal

☐ C Arterial P_{O_2} is normal or high

☐ D Haemoglobin releases oxygen less readily in the tissues

☐ E Most likely diagnosis is COPD

3.15 **A 50-year-old man is brought to hospital by ambulance complaining of increasing breathlessness. You perform arterial blood gases, which reveal type II respiratory failure. What is the most likely diagnosis?**

☐ A Sarcoidosis

☐ B Fibrosing alveolitis

☐ C Myasthenia gravis

☐ D Salicylate poisoning

☐ E Extrinsic allergic alveolitis

3.16 **A 63-year-old woman is referred to your clinic with increasing breathlessness. She has previously had a 50 pack/year smoking history. She appears hyperinflated and you think she probably has COPD/emphysema. Which one of the following statements concerning COPD/emphysema is correct?**

- ☐ A Compliance is reduced
- ☐ B Emphysematous changes in the lower lobes suggest α_1-antitrypsin deficiency
- ☐ C Paradoxical downward movement of the diaphragm with inspiration is seen due to downward movement of the costal margin
- ☐ D Cardiac arrhythmias are uncommon
- ☐ E Functional dead space decreases

3.17 **A 67-year-old man has a chest X-ray performed for an insurance medical. There is evidence of bilateral pleural calcification. Which one of the following is the most likely diagnosis?**

- ☐ A Occupational asbestos exposure
- ☐ B Haemothorax
- ☐ C Tuberculous pleural effusion
- ☐ D Previous empyema
- ☐ E Chickenpox pneumonia

3.18 **A 30-year-old African man is admitted to hospital with fever, cough and night sweats. The admitting team seek your specialist opinion because they think he may have miliary tuberculosis. Which one of the following statements regarding military tuberculosis is correct?**

- ☐ A A normal chest X-ray excludes the diagnosis
- ☐ B A negative tuberculin test excludes the diagnosis
- ☐ C Anti-TB drugs are not indicated unless sputum is positive for acid-fast bacilli
- ☐ D Nodules are characteristically 3–5 mm in diameter
- ☐ E Tuberculous meningitis co-exists in about a third of patients

3.19 **A nurse on the ward becomes concerned because a patient has an oxygen saturation (SpO$_2$) of 92% whilst breathing room air. You explain to her about how this relates to arterial Po$_2$. Which one of the following statements regarding the oxygen-haemoglobin dissociation curve is true?**

- ☐ A   Myoglobin shifts the curve to the right
- ☐ B   Decreased pH shifts the curve to the left (Bohr effect)
- ☐ C   The curve has a sigmoid shape due to varying affinities of the globin groups for oxygen
- ☐ D   A shift to the left increases the slope of the curve because affinity of haemoglobin for oxygen has been decreased
- ☐ E   Arterial blood Po$_2$ (95 mmHg/12.4 kPa) is less than alveolar Po$_2$ because of arterio-venous shunting

3.20 **You are performing an audit of asthma management in your Emergency Department. Whilst doing this one of the doctors asks you to explain how all the asthma drugs work. Which one of the following statements regarding asthma therapy is true?**

- ☐ A   Smoking increases the clearance of theophylline
- ☐ B   Anticholinergic drugs are more effective than β-agonists in acute asthma
- ☐ C   Acute asthma is typically associated with hyperkalaemia
- ☐ D   Steroids stimulate the formation of cytokines by lymphocytes and macrophages
- ☐ E   Montelukast is best taken prior to exercise in adults with exercise-induced asthma

3.21 **A 36-year-old breathless woman is referred with possible pulmonary hypertension. Which one of the following is true concerning her diagnosis and management?**

- ☐ A   It is associated with a split second heart sound
- ☐ B   It may be diagnosed from a mean pulmonary artery pressure above 25 mmHg on exercise
- ☐ C   The primary disease affects men more than women
- ☐ D   Adenosine via pulmonary artery catheter may be used as an acute vasodilator
- ☐ E   Pulmonary vascular resistance falls with severe disease

3.22 A 49-year-old man with a body mass index of 38 kg/m^2 is referred because of snoring. He comes to the clinic with his wife, a GP practice nurse, who tells you that his snoring wakes up the neighbours and that he seems to stop breathing several times per night. She is concerned that he may have obstructive sleep apnoea. Which one of the following features is he least likely to have if his wife has the correct diagnosis?

☐ A Systemic hypertension

☐ B Pulmonary hypertension

☐ C Daytime insomnolence

☐ D Polycythaemia

☐ E Depression

3.23 A 74-year-old man who has smoked all his life presents with haemoptysis and weight loss. Bronchoscopy reveals the presence of a malignant neoplasm of the lung. Which one of the following is true concerning his possible treatment for his lung cancer?

☐ A Limited-disease small-cell carcinoma should be treated with eight cycles of combination chemotherapy

☐ B Adriamycin may cause a peripheral neuropathy

☐ C In small-cell lung carcinoma mediastinal irradiation should be given prior to chemotherapy

☐ D Hypertrophic pulmonary osteoarthropathy (HPOA) can resolve if the primary tumour is treated

☐ E Elderly patients are unable to tolerate chemotherapy or surgery and should receive palliative care only

3.24   A 61-year-old man with an 80 pack/year smoking history is flagged up by your radiologist with an abnormal chest X-ray. The patient's GP had sent him for this investigation because of chronic cough. The chest X-ray shows a mass in the right lower zone and bronchoscopic washings from the right lower lobe yields malignant cells. Blood tests are abnormal and you consider the possibility of a paraneoplastic phenomenon. Which one of the following is true concerning paraneoplastic phenomena?

- [ ] A   Cushing's syndrome may be due to ectopic ACTH secretion
- [ ] B   Eaton–Lambert syndrome occurs most commonly with small-cell carcinoma
- [ ] C   Desmopressin is used to correct hyponatraemia in the syndrome of inappropriate antidiuretic hormone secretion (SIADH)
- [ ] D   Hypercalcaemia in lung cancer is most commonly due to ectopic parathormone (PTH) secretion
- [ ] E   The presence of a paraneoplastic syndrome is a contraindication to surgery

3.25   A 43-year-old man consults you as he is producing a cupful of foul purulent sputum every day. Examination reveals digital clubbing and coarse crackles at the left base. What is the most likely diagnosis?

- [ ] A   Bronchiectasis
- [ ] B   Acute lung abscess
- [ ] C   Bronchoalveolar cell carcinoma (BAC)
- [ ] D   Fibrosing alveolitis
- [ ] E   Sarcoidosis

3.26   A 36-year-old, non-smoking lady presents to the Emergency Department with a complete spontaneous right-sided pneumothorax. This is treated with chest drainage and a chest X-ray then shows diffuse reticular shadowing in both lung fields. On further questioning she admits to worsening breathlessness over several years and a previous right-sided pneumothorax. Which one of the following diagnoses is the most appropriate?

- [ ] A   Churg–Strauss vasculitis
- [ ] B   Cryptogenic organising pneumonia
- [ ] C   Langerhans' cell histiocytosis
- [ ] D   Lymphangioleiomyomatosis
- [ ] E   Sarcoidosis

3.27 An 85-year-old lady with haemoptysis presents to Respiratory Outpatients with a large mass in the right lung on her chest X-ray and an enlarged paratracheal lymph node. She is found to have an FEV_1 of 0.8 l and an O_2 saturation of 90% on air. Which one of the following would be the most appropriate method of diagnosis in such a patient?

- ☐ A   Bronchoscopy
- ☐ B   Mediastinoscopy
- ☐ C   Percutaneous biopsy
- ☐ D   Positron emission tomography
- ☐ E   Sputum cytology

3.28 An 18-year-old previously fit and well student is admitted to the Emergency Department with worsening breathlessness. Chest X-ray reveals a complete right-sided pneumothorax. There is no history of chest trauma. His observations are stable and he has saturations of 95% on air. Which one of the following interventions is the most appropriate in this clinical setting?

- ☐ A   Analgesia and observation
- ☐ B   Chest drain and negative-pressure suction
- ☐ C   Large-bore chest drain insertion
- ☐ D   Pleural aspiration alone
- ☐ E   Small-bore chest drain insertion

3.29 A 45-year-old lady with breast carcinoma attends the Emergency Department with a history of rapid onset of chest pain and breathlessness since arriving at Heathrow Airport earlier in the day after a long-haul flight back from seeing family in Australia. She is tachypnoeic, tachycardic and hypotensive. Which one of the following investigations would you perform first to make the diagnosis of pulmonary embolism (PE)?

- ☐ A   Echocardiography
- ☐ B   Leg Doppler ultrasound
- ☐ C   Serum D-dimer
- ☐ D   Spiral CT scanning
- ☐ E   V/Q scanning

3.30 A 60-year-old man has been followed up in the Chest Clinic for several months for recurrent episodes of breathlessness associated with bilateral opacification on chest X-ray. Over a period of weeks each episode slowly resolves. He is a smoker and keeps two budgies at home in the front room. Which one of the following lung disorders would be the most likely diagnosis in this case?

- ☐ A Cryptogenic organising pneumonia (COP)
- ☐ B Extrinsic allergic alveolitis (EAA)
- ☐ C Langerhans' cell histiocytosis
- ☐ D Sarcoidosis
- ☐ E Wegener's granulomatosis

3.31 Which one of the following organisms is least likely to cause severe community-acquired pneumonia (CAP)?

- ☐ A Gram-negative *Enterobacteriaceae*
- ☐ B *Legionella pneumophila*
- ☐ C *Mycoplasma pneumoniae*
- ☐ D *Staphylococcus aureus*
- ☐ E *Streptococcus pneumoniae*

3.32 Pneumonia in the immunocompromised host is caused by a host of pathogens. Which one of the following statements is most likely to be false?

- ☐ A Immunecompromise associated with bone marrow transplantation is closely associated with cytomegalovirus pneumonitis
- ☐ B Pneumonia in the immunocompromised host with B cell dysfunction is commonly associated with a bacterial aetiology
- ☐ C *Streptococcus pneumoniae* is an unlikely pathogen in pneumonia associated with HIV infection
- ☐ D T cell dysfunction may be associated with pneumonia due to intracellular pathogens and opportunistic infections
- ☐ E The most likely pathogen causing pneumonia in HIV infection with CD4 counts < 200 is *Pneumocystis carinii*

3.33   **In suspected *Legionella pneumophila* pneumonia, which one of the following diagnostic tests would be most likely to confirm the diagnosis in the acute setting?**

☐   A   Acute serology

☐   B   Blood culture

☐   C   Sputum culture

☐   D   Sputum Gram stain

☐   E   Urinary antigen testing

3.34   **A pregnant woman consults you because of mild breathlessness, which she thinks may be a pulmonary embolism. You successfully exclude this possibility and also exclude any significant respiratory pathology. However, she asks you if pregnancy can cause any physiological pulmonary alterations. Which one of the following physiological explanations concerning the respiratory system in pregnancy is false?**

☐   A   A mild compensated respiratory alkalosis develops

☐   B   Functional residual capacity (FRC) decreases by approximately 25%

☐   C   Oxygen requirements increase by approximately 30–40 ml/min

☐   D   Tidal volume increases by approximately 40%

☐   E   Total pulmonary compliance is increased

3.35   **A 35-year-old man who smokes 20 cigarettes per day develops emphysema. Further questioning reveals that his father had emphysema at a similar young age. You check his α_1-antitrypsin genotype and find him to be a PiZZ homozygote. What is his approximate α_1-antitrypsin level likely to be?**

☐   A   100% of normal

☐   B   75% of normal

☐   C   50% of normal

☐   D   30% of normal

☐   E   15% of normal

3.36   **Which one of the following treatments is the most important and effective for acute anaphylaxis (eg to drugs or insect envenomation)?**

☐   A   0.5 ml adrenaline 1:1000 intramuscularly

☐   B   10 ml adrenaline 1:10, 000 intravenously

☐   C   Intravenous antihistamines

☐   D   Intravenous antihistamines and intravenous hydrocortisone

☐   E   5 ml adrenaline 1:1000 subcutaneously

3.37   **A 25-year-old man is seen in the TB Contact Clinic because his wife has sputum smear-positive pulmonary TB. The TB clinic has run out of Heaf test reagent and the nurse therefore calls you to insert a Mantoux test. What dose of Mantoux would you insert?**

☐   A   1 ml of 1:100 intradermally

☐   B   0.1 ml of 1:10, 000 subcutaneously

☐   C   1 ml of 1:1000 intradermally

☐   D   0.1 ml 1:1000 intradermally

☐   E   1 ml of 1:100 subcutaneously

3.38   **A patient with known Churg–Strauss syndrome is admitted with an acute exacerbation. His lung function tests show him to have a gas transfer factor (TLCO) of 50% predicted. Which of the following combinations of % predicted transfer coefficient (KCO) and alveolar volume (VA) are most likely to account for the abnormal TLCO in this patient?**

☐   A   VA 35   KCO 130

☐   B   VA 45   KCO 120

☐   C   VA 50   KCO 100

☐   D   VA 70   KCO 70

☐   E   VA 100 KCO 50

3.39 **A 78-year-old man with severe COPD (FEV$_1$ 0.8 litres) has been housebound for three years. His GP requests his admission to hospital, as the patient is confused and breathless. His arterial blood gases on 24% O$_2$ show PaO$_2$ 5.3 kPa (~40 mmHg), PaCO$_2$ 9.2 kPa (~70 mmHg) with a normal pH. You increase his inspired oxygen to 28% and repeat blood gases show PaO$_2$ 7.3 kPa (~55 mmHg) and PaCO$_2$ 10.5 kPa (~80 mmHg) but he has become acidotic. What would your next management step be?**

- ☐ A Bi-level positive airway pressure (BiPAP)
- ☐ B Check resuscitation status with next of kin
- ☐ C Continuous positive airway pressure (CPAP)
- ☐ D Immediate endotracheal intubation and mechanical ventilation
- ☐ E Intravenous doxapram

3.40 **A 52-year-old man with newly diagnosed cryptogenic fibrosing alveolitis asks you about his long-term prognosis and likely response to treatment. Which of the following is most likely to predict a good response to corticosteroids?**

- ☐ A Absence of pulmonary hypertension on transthoracic echocardiography
- ☐ B Bronchoalveolar lavage (BAL) lymphocytosis
- ☐ C PaO$_2$ > 8.0 kPa (60 mmHg) on air
- ☐ D Predominant reticular pattern on high-resolution computed tomography (HRCT)
- ☐ E Rapid diethylene-triamine-penta-acetic acid (DTPA) clearance

3.41 **A 60-year-old man who has a history of heavy asbestos exposure in the past comes to your clinic because of progressive breathlessness. His lung function tests show decreased spirometric lung volumes with a forced expiratory ratio of 80%. His gas transfer factor (TLco) is 55% of predicted and transfer coefficient (Kco) is 60% of predicted. What is the most likely explanation for these abnormalities?**

- ☐ A Asbestos-induced bronchial carcinoma
- ☐ B Asbestos plaques
- ☐ C Asbestosis
- ☐ D Diffuse pleural thickening secondary to asbestos
- ☐ E Malignant mesothelioma

3.42   **A 35-year-old Afro-Caribbean man comes to your clinic with a letter from a physician he consulted whilst in the USA for several months. This letter explains that he has sarcoidosis and some investigations are appended. Which of the following results would be an indication for systemic corticosteroid treatment?**

☐ A   Arterial blood gases showing PaO$_2$ on air of 9.2 kPa (70 mmHg)

☐ B   Bilateral hilar lymphadenopathy on chest X-ray

☐ C   Evidence of ground-glass opacification on high-resolution CT thorax

☐ D   Gas transfer factor (TLco) of 75% predicted

☐ E   24-hour urinary calcium of 12 mmol/l

3.43   **A 45-year-old computer engineer presents to you with breathlessness. At home he has an aviary with parrots, budgerigars and parakeets. He has read on the Internet that his exposure to these birds might lead to the development of extrinsic allergic alveolitis (EAA). Which one of the following tests is most likely to help you decide whether he has EAA?**

☐ A   CT thorax with 2-mm slices

☐ B   CT thorax with 10-mm slices

☐ C   DTPA scanning

☐ D   Magnetic resonance imaging (MRI) thorax

☐ E   Positron emission tomography (PET) scan of thorax

3.44   **A 32-year-old woman with systemic sclerosis is referred to you by your local rheumatologist because of progressive breathlessness. The referral letter says that she is anti-topoisomerase I (Scl-70) antibody-positive. Which of the following is most likely to be the cause of her breathlessness?**

☐ A   Fibrosing alveolitis

☐ B   Organising pneumonia

☐ C   Pulmonary vascular disease

☐ D   Recurrent pulmonary aspiration

☐ E   Shrinking lung due to pleural involvement

3.45 A 60-year-old man with a smoking history of 40/day over many years has a chest X-ray because of breathlessness. This shows a solitary ill-defined mass in the left lower lobe, which on bronchoscopic biopsy turns out to be a squamous cell carcinoma. Which of the following features would render this patient's tumour inoperable?

☐ A FEV_1 of 1.6 litres

☐ B   Hypercalcaemia

☐ C   Ipsilateral mediastinal lymph node metastasis

☐ D   Ipsilateral supraclavicular lymph node metastasis

☐ E   Pleural effusion

3.46 In a patient with smoking-related chronic obstructive pulmonary disease (COPD), which of the following is true regarding indications for long-term oxygen therapy (LTOT).

☐ A   Exercise tolerance of less than 100 metres on a flat road

☐ B   Forced expiratory ratio of less than 65%

☐ C FEV_1 less than 1.5 litres

☐ D   Gas transfer factor (T_{LCO}) of less than 65% predicted

☐ E Pao_2 less than 8.5 kPa (~ 65 mmHg)

3.47 A 45-year-old man is referred to you because of breathlessness. You diagnose a pleural effusion, which you aspirate and find to have an eosinophilia. Which of the following diagnoses is least likely?

☐ A   Asbestos pleural effusion

☐ B   Drug reaction

☐ C   Fungal infection

☐ D   Haemopneumothorax

☐ E   Malignant pleural effusion

3.48   A 35-year-old man has a chest X-ray as part of a routine employment medical. A mass is seen and, with the help of a lateral film, is seen to be in the anterior mediastinum. Which of the following is the least likely diagnosis?

☐   A   Dermoid cyst

☐   B   Hernia of the foramen of Morgagni

☐   C   Hodgkin's lymphoma

☐   D   Leiomyoma of the oesophagus

☐   E   Malignant thymoma

3.49   You are called to see a 26-year-old man on the Intensive Care Unit following an inhalational injury. The nursing staff are concerned he may be developing acute respiratory distress syndrome (ARDS). Which one of the following features would be consistent with ARDS?

☐   A   Elevation in gas transfer coefficient (K_{CO})

☐   B   Increase in lung compliance

☐   C   Increase in lung elastic recoil

☐   D Pao_2:Fio_2 ratio of 350 mmHg

☐   E   Pulmonary capillary wedge pressure of 30 mmHg

3.50   A 35-year-old man with fever, cough and night sweats is found to have pulmonary tuberculosis. Which of the following statements regarding management is correct?

☐   A   All patients should be managed in a negative-pressure ventilation room

☐   B   Corticosteroids are contraindicated

☐   C   Ethambutol should not be used in patients who wear glasses for myopia

☐   D   Multidrug-resistant TB (MDRTB) requires the addition of two or more drugs at a time in a failing regimen

☐   E   Rifampicin and isoniazid must not be used if the patient is HIV-positive

CARDIOLOGY: 'BEST OF FIVE' ANSWERS

1.1   E: Increased splitting of the second heart sound

During inspiration the intrathoracic pressure decreases, so that blood is drawn into the lung vessels. As a result blood is sucked through the right side of the heart into the lungs, but prevented from flowing out of the pulmonary veins into the systemic circulation. The right atrial and systemic arterial pressures decrease and heart rate increases. The increased blood flow through the right ventricle and decreased flow through the left ventricle means that pulmonary valve closure is delayed and aortic valve closure is earlier, which exaggerates the normal splitting of the second heart sound. The jugular venous pressure falls, heart rate increases and systemic blood pressure decreases. Diastolic murmurs are always pathological.

1.2   A: Inotropic support

If an isolated right ventricular infarct is suspected fluid resuscitation is indicated. However, at a wedge pressure of 20 mmHg the patient is teetering on the brink of pulmonary oedema. In cardiogenic shock the blood pressure should be raised before furosemide is given. There is nothing in the history to suggest that rescue angioplasty is required although this would be preferred to repeat thrombolysis if re-perfusion were indicated. Resuscitation should be commenced before any intravascular procedure.

1.3   D: Calcium ions are required for electromechanical coupling of the cardiac myosite

Cardiac muscle contracts rhythmically, unlike other forms of muscle. However, like other types of muscle the myocardial cells depolarise as a result of sodium influx and repolarise because of potassium efflux. The plateau phase is caused by calcium influx. Electromechanical coupling is dependent on calcium ions and adenosine triphosphate (ATP). ATP is the energy source for myocardial cells.

1.4   D: VVI pacing

In the jugular venous pressure waveform the *a* wave corresponds to atrial contraction. The *v* wave is caused by the final phase of atrial filling, the descending limb of the *v* wave (the *y* descent) is caused by ventricular filling as the tricuspid valve opens. In contrast to the physiological state, in tricuspid regurgitation the *v* wave corresponds to ventricular contraction and therefore occurs simultaneously with the carotid pulse. As such it truly represents a *cv* wave. Cannon waves are due to simultaneous ventricular and atrial contraction and may occur with VVI pacing or complete heart block. The associated rise in left atrial pressure and reduction in ventricular filling is the cause of the pacemaker syndrome. Constrictive and restrictive cardiac disease, along with tamponade, cause paradoxical increase in jugular venous pressure on inspiration. In atrial fibrillation the *a* wave is lost.

1.5   C: Vasodilatation in response to acetylcholine

Endothelial-derived relaxation factor (nitric oxide, NO) is produced by endothelial cells from L-arginine in response to ischaemia. Nitrates are NO-releasing compounds augmenting this production. NO is a potent vasodilator which also inhibits platelet adhesion and aggregation. NO treats angina by causing vasodilatation through acetylcholine release. This dilates coronary arteries and reduces pre-load and afterload. Endothelin is a peptide released in response to endothelial damage which acts as a vasoconstrictor and promotes smooth muscle cell mitogenesis and proliferation.

1.6   D: Massive pulmonary embolism

Pulsus paradoxus is an exaggeration of the normal slight fall in arterial pressure that occurs during inspiration and rises during expiration. Pulsus paradoxus occurs when greater than normal negative intrathoracic pressures are generated during inspiration (eg asthma). When positive pressure ventilation is used, intrathoracic pressure is raised during inspiration so that blood pressure rises. Left ventricular underfilling is an important requirement for pulsus paradoxus and occurs in hypovolaemia and massive pulmonary embolism. Pulsus paradoxus also occurs in patients with cardiac tamponade, but when valvular lesions (eg aortic regurgitation) which prevent left ventricular underfilling are also present, pulsus paradoxus does not occur. In advanced heart failure pulsus alternans sometimes occurs.

1.7   D: Pre-systolic accentuation of the diastolic murmur occurs if the patient is in sinus rhythm

The first sound and the opening snap become softer as the valve calcifies and becomes rigid. The opening snap gets earlier as the disease progresses because the left atrial pressure rises and thus exceeds left ventricular pressure earlier in diastole. Pre-systolic accentuation of the diastolic murmur is due to atrial contraction, so it disappears with the onset of atrial fibrillation. The early diastolic murmur described by Graham Steell is due to pulmonary regurgitation. Mitral stenosis is three to four times more common in women than in men.

1.8   A: Familial hyperalphalipoproteinaemia

Familial hyperalphalipoproteinaemia is due to an increased production of HDL which protects against atheromatous coronary disease. Familial mixed hyperlipidaemia is found in 15% of patients with coronary artery disease who are under 60. It is associated with an increase in LDL and triglyceride levels. Hormone replacement therapy in post-menopausal women has been shown to reduce the risk of coronary events. This effect is due to oestrogen supplementation which lowers LDL and increases HDL levels. These effects are partly antagonised by progestogens in the combined preparations. Familial hypercholesterolaemia affects 0.2% of the population; both heterozygous and homozygous forms are associated with coronary artery disease. Hypothyroidism is associated with an increase in serum cholesterol and triglycerides.

1.9   B: The first heart sound and the onset of the carotid upstroke

Left ventricular isovolumic contraction occurs between closure of the mitral valve (first heart sound) and opening of the aortic valve (carotid upstroke). The jugular *a* wave corresponds to atrial systole and the *v* wave to atrial filling: both occur in ventricular diastole. The third and fourth heart sounds also occur in ventricular diastole and are the result of passive and then active filling of the ventricle. The second heart sound marks the end of ventricular systole and the interval between aortic and pulmonary components increases in inspiration.

1.10   A: Captopril

ACE inhibitors have been shown to reduce mortality post-myocardial infarction (MI) in a number of studies. In the ISIS-4 trial captopril was used in all patients post-MI and was shown to reduce mortality by 7%. This survival advantage was maintained at a year. In the same trial nitrates were shown to be ineffective. The TRENT study found that nifedipine increased mortality post-MI. Nicorandil has shown a trend toward mortality reduction in stable angina. Other proven drugs in secondary prevention are anti-platelet agents, β-blockers and statins.

1.11   D: Oligaemic lung fields on chest X-ray

The features of Fallot's tetralogy are due to a combination of a ventricular septal defect and pulmonary stenosis. This causes shunting of blood from the right to left ventricles, which results in cyanosis. However, in mild cases, cyanosis does not develop until a day or two after birth, when the ductus arteriosus closes. The presence of the right-to-left shunt also causes diversion of blood away from the lungs, which appear oligaemic on chest X-ray and can result in paradoxical emboli, eg clots in deep veins of the legs can pass to the left circulation and cause embolic CVA. The presence of pulmonary stenosis protects against development of pulmonary hypertension. The second heart sound is single.

1.12   E: β-Blocker therapy

ST segment changes on a resting ECG due to left ventricular hypertrophy or dilatation make the interpretation of the ETT difficult. In these cases the use of thallium-201 imaging in combination with exercise may improve the diagnostic yield. Exercise testing in aortic stenosis is hazardous and should be undertaken with caution. Left bundle branch block (LBBB) makes interpretation of ECG changes impossible, but the development of LBBB at heart rates greater than 125 bpm in the absence of chest pain is not associated with coronary artery disease. Patients on β-blockers often have false negative exercise tests, making the investigation less sensitive but not affecting specificity.

1.13   D: Associated with an increased incidence of bicuspid aortic valve

A coarctation is a narrowing or obliteration of the aortic lumen. It may be acquired but is usually congenital, when it is most commonly situated just distal to the origin of the left subclavian artery. Coarctation of the aorta is the commonest cause of heart failure in babies who are not cyanosed and is an uncommon cause of hypertension in adult life. Coarctation is associated with other cardiac abnormalities, particularly bicuspid aortic valve, but does not itself cause cardiac shunting. Coarctation is recognised by absent or delayed pulses in the legs compared with those in the arms.

1.14   A: The risk of embolic stroke is increased fivefold

Non-rheumatic atrial fibrillation (AF) is associated with a fivefold risk of embolic stroke compared with a 15-fold risk for rheumatic AF. Excessive alcohol intake is a common cause. Other causes include hypertension, ischaemic heart disease, thyrotoxicosis and pulmonary embolic disease. Paroxysmal AF carries the same risk of stroke as continuous AF. Cardioversion may be performed without prior anticoagulation in patients with a normal transoesophageal echocardiogram. A normal transthoracic echo does not exclude the presence of left atrial thrombus. Anticoagulation is required for up to four weeks after cardioversion.

1.15   C: The law means that stroke volume is proportional to left ventricular end-diastolic volume unless the inotropic state of the myocardium or vascular resistance change

Starling's law states that in the isolated heart the force of contraction is directly proportional to the initial length of the cardiac fibre. When extrapolated to the whole animal, contractility and output impedance are also important determinants of stroke volume. However, factors which reduce cardiac filling generally also reduce stroke volume, but do not necessarily alter contractility. The law is dependent on the properties of myosites and the actin-myosin interaction. The cardiac stretch receptors do not play any part in Starling's law.

1.16   D: The patient has a conduction disturbance in their normal rhythm

During ventricular tachycardia the atria continue their own independent activity, unless retrograde activation of the atria is occurring through the atrioventricular node. Evidence of atrial activity independent of the ventricular tachycardia includes cannon waves (when atria and ventricles coincidentally contract simultaneously), atrioventricular dissociation and fusion beats on the ECG. Supraventricular tachycardia (SVT) is quite often abolished by carotid sinus massage but ventricular tachycardia is not. When the pattern of ventricular activation during the tachycardia is the same as sometimes occurs during sinus rhythm, this strongly suggests the presence of supraventricular tachycardia with aberrant conduction. Most ventricular tachycardias are of right bundle morphology.

1.17   E: Pulmonary oedema due to mitral stenosis in pregnancy is usually best treated by valvotomy

During pregnancy cardiac output increases and new murmurs are usually innocent flow murmurs. However, a cardiomyopathy is well described in association with pregnancy, and pre-existing cardiac lesions are more likely to present at this time of increased cardiac work. Mitral stenosis requiring intervention during pregnancy is usually treated by valvotomy. Use of anticoagulants in pregnant women (or young women who may subsequently become pregnant) does present problems. Oral anticoagulants are teratogenic and can cross the placenta with the risk of placental and fetal haemorrhage.

1.18   A: Stimulation of the carotid sinus and aortic baroreceptors by a reduced blood pressure

On standing from the supine position, blood pools in the venous capacitance vessels of the legs. Cardiac output falls and total peripheral resistance increases. The arterial pressure at the level of the arterial baroreceptors is reduced and this stimulates compensatory changes. Homoeostatic mechanisms include increased angiotensin II secretion and sympathetic stimulation. On standing, the arterial pressure in the cerebral vessels is reduced because these are now the highest part of the body. Cerebral blood flow is reduced and, as a result, the P_{CO_2} in brain tissue increases and the P_{O_2} decreases. These changes stimulate autoregulation of cerebral blood flow.

1.19   E: Bisoprolol and warfarin

With intermittent atrial fibrillaton, ischaemic heart disease and impaired ventricular function, this man will benefit from full anticoagulation to reduce stroke risk. With impaired ventricular function and ischaemic heart disease he will benefit from β-blockade. It would be logical to start anticoagulation and β-blocking agents. Although amiodarone is an acceptable answer from the anti-arrhythmic perspective it ignores the prognostic benefit this man will derive from β-blockade and is not offered as an answer in conjunction with anticoagulation. Flecainide and sotalol are associated with excess mortality in patients with ischaemia or heart failure. Digoxin limits ventricular rate in sustained AF but does not reduce episodes of intermittent AF.

1.20   E: The cardiovascular responses to the manoeuvre may be blunted in diabetes

The Valsalva manoeuvre is performed by forced expiration against a closed glottis. The initial increase in intrathoracic pressure causes blood pressure to increase, but this soon falls because venous return is impaired. The fall in blood pressure is accompanied by a tachycardia and a rise in peripheral vascular resistance which are mediated through the baroreceptors. On release of the manoeuvre, venous return increases and hence blood pressure increases and in fact overshoots normal. This hypertension is accompanied by bradycardia. These cardiovascular effects persist after sympathectomy because the baroreceptors and vagi are intact. The responses can be impaired when autonomic neuropathy is present (eg in some diabetics).

1.21 C: β-Blockade may result in symptomatic improvement in cases of dilated cardiomyopathy

ACE inhibitors were shown in the CONSENSUS I study to reduce mortality in patients with severe cardiac failure by 40%. Dihydropyridines such as nifedipine are not associated with any mortality benefit and may be detrimental. In the Veterans Administration study a combination of hydralazine and nitrates was shown to improve survival, but this was pre-β-blockers and other studies have cast doubt on the value and safety of vasodilating agents. Careful introduction of low-dose β-blockade improves symptoms and prognosis in patients with dilated cardiomyopathy. Digoxin is an accepted treatment in patients with left ventricular failure in sinus rhythm. A third sound is associated with filling of a non-compliant left ventricle.

1.22 A: Peripheral vascular resistance rises

After birth, the lungs inflate which causes pulmonary vascular resistance to fall. In utero, the placental vessels cause the systemic vascular resistance to be low and inferior vena caval flow to be high. When placental blood flow ceases, the systemic vascular resistance rises and for the first time superior vena caval flow exceeds inferior vena caval flow. Also at birth the foramen ovale closes (rather like a flap) as left atrial pressure and lung blood flow increase. The ductus arteriosus narrows at birth but does not close for a day or two. During those initial days, the direction of flow across the ductus arteriosus is reversed since the high pulmonary vascular resistance and low systemic vascular resistance present in utero are reversed.

1.23 E: They usually arise from a pedicle near to the fossa ovalis

Atrial myxomas usually arise near to the fossa ovalis. They are twice as common in the left atrium as in the right. They cause valve dysfunction, emboli, fever, joint pains, a raised ESR and anaemia. Thus the findings are often similar to those of infective endocarditis. The tumours are well visualised on echocardiography. After resection the tumour may recur, particularly if any part of the pedicle is not removed.

1.24 B: Marked ST elevation with increased R wave amplitude was present during anginal attacks

Prinzmetal's angina is angina at rest with ST-segment elevation. It is felt to be due to coronary artery spasm. Some 60–70% of patients have severe proximal coronary atherosclerosis. Ventricular arrhythmias occur in about 50% of patients during pain and may be responsible for syncope. A fifth of patients with Prinzmetal's angina have a myocardial infarction within six months of presentation. A, C, D and E are all associations but B is the defining feature and is therefore the best answer.

1.25   D: Increased circulating renin concentrations

Neither the basal metabolic rate nor the oxygen carrying capacity of the blood is altered in congestive heart failure. Instead, responses to reductions in blood pressure and cardiac output occur as if these were due to hypovolaemia. The resulting homoeostatic mechanisms are designed to increase circulating volume by retaining salt and water as well as to raise blood pressure by vasoconstriction and inotropic stimulation of the heart. Changes include increased renin secretion and inappropriate aldosterone secretion (ie normal or raised aldosterone despite sodium retention). Circulating catecholamines are raised but cardiac responsiveness is decreased, possibly due to receptor down-regulation

1.26   B: ACE inhibitor

While all of these agents are effective antihypertensives, an angiotensin-converting-enzyme (ACE) inhibitor, if tolerated, would be the optimal initial therapeutic option in a patient with prior coronary artery bypass grafting (CABG). In addition to their beneficial effects on blood pressure reduction, ACE inhibitors appear to have additional benefits in patients with evidence of significant vascular disease, irrespective of left ventricular function. The HOPE study demonstrated that treatment with ramipril reduced the rates of death, myocardial infarction and stroke to an extent that could not be accounted for by blood pressure reduction alone. This study included patients with known angina, previous unstable angina, percutaneous coronary intervention and CABG.

1.27   D: Troponin I level

A plasma troponin I measured 12 hours after symptoms would be extremely helpful in determining this patient's initial management. If this is negative and the ECG normal, then it is safe to send the patient home and arrange further investigations as an outpatient, if required. Plasma levels of troponin I are highly specific for myocardial damage, and in particular a normal level measured at 12 hours has a very high negative predictive value for adverse cardiac events in the context of a normal ECG. Plasma levels can, however, be elevated in renal failure. Although an exercise test would also help clarify diagnosis and subsequent risk, this should not be performed until cardiac enzymes have excluded an acute cardiac event in patients presenting with significant chest pain. Clearly, if diagnostic doubt still exists or an exercise test is positive, angiography would be warranted.

1.28   C: Thrombolysis with streptokinase

Although this lady has developed CHB she is haemodynamically stable, without clinical evidence of pulmonary oedema. This has occurred in the context of an acute inferior infarction, primarily because the right coronary artery contributes to the blood supply of the atrioventricular (AV) node (via the AV nodal branch). In acute myocardial infarction early restoration of coronary artery blood flow has a major influence on prognosis. In a 70-year-old lady with an inferior infarct this would usually be attempted with thrombolysis in the form of streptokinase. Although temporary pacing has not been shown to improve prognosis in acute myocardial infarction, it should be used in patients with inferior infarction and CHB with evidence of haemodynamic compromise.

Patients presenting with CHB in the context of an anterior infarct have a particularly poor prognosis, primarily due to the extensive amount of damaged myocardium. In this situation temporary pacing should be routinely used to try to prevent bradycardia-associated hypotension and the increased risk of ventricular asystole associated with this presentation.

1.29   C: Presence of co-existing coronary artery disease

Symptomatic aortic stenosis is an indication for surgery (unless determined inappropriate for other medical reasons). Transthoracic echocardiography can provide accurate details of peak aortic valve gradient together with estimates of left ventricular function. Patients with evidence of left ventricular dysfunction, even if severe, should still undergo assessment for valve replacement since function may significantly improve post-operatively and prognosis without surgery is particularly poor. It is, however, important to know about the coronary anatomy in the majority of cases: this will determine the requirement for concomitant coronary artery bypass grafting and peri-operative risk. Right heart pressures will not influence the need for surgical intervention and although there may be co-existent aortic incompetence there is no doubt in this case that valve replacement is required.

1.30   A: Addition of β-blocker

There is now considerable evidence to support the use of β-blockers in the treatment of chronic heart failure for patients in either sinus rhythm or AF (COPERNICUS – carvedilol, CBIS-II – bisoprolol, MERIT-HF – metoprolol). Although digoxin is usually effective in controlling resting heart rates it is not as good at controlling increased rates occurring during exercise. β-blockers are, however, particularly useful in this setting. AV node ablation and pacemaker insertion is an irreversible intervention and should be reserved for patients intolerant of medication or in whom it is ineffective despite adequate dosing. AF can be paroxysmal, persistent (but possibly amenable to cardioversion) or permanent. By definition, permanent AF cannot be converted to sinus rhythm.

1.31   C: Radiofrequency ablation of the accessory pathway

The history is suggestive of paroxysmal AF in the context of WPW. In WPW the ventricular response during AF can be extremely rapid as a result of anterograde conduction down the accessory pathway. This can degenerate into ventricular fibrillation. In this young, symptomatic patient radiofrequency ablation of the accessory pathway is a potentially curative procedure that can be carried out with minimal risk. Although treatment with amiodarone, flecainide or sotalol might be effective in reducing or even abolishing symptoms, therapy would need to be maintained long-term.

1.32   B: Constrictive pericarditis

In constrictive pericarditis the heavily fibrosed or calcified pericardium restricts diastolic filling of all four chambers of the heart. Patients often present with dyspnoea and fatigue together with symptoms and signs of marked fluid retention. In this case pericardial constriction could be a result of previous tuberculous pericarditis or be secondary to radiotherapy. Examination of the JVP can be very helpful in the clinical assessment of pericardial disease. In constrictive pericarditis there is a rapid *y* descent, since the majority of ventricular filling occurs in early diastole. Kussmaul's sign (an increase in systemic venous pressure during inspiration) is also seen and results from a failure of transmission of the intra-thoracic pressure changes to the pericardial space, seen during normal respiration. In cardiac tamponade the *y* descent is often absent or blunted. Severe tricuspid incompetence is associated with giant *v* waves whereas in superior vena cava obstruction the JVP is elevated and fixed. Patients with tamponade typically demonstrate a significant degree of pulsus parodoxus (> 10 mmHg), whereas in those with constriction this tends to occur to a lesser degree (< 10 mmHg).

1.33   B: ASD – ostium secundum

The results show normal aortic and wedge pressures but slightly elevated right heart pressures. A step-up in saturation is seen at the level of the right atrium, thereby demonstrating the presence of a left-to-right shunt at this level and thus confirming the diagnosis of an atrial septal defect. Secundum defects are the most common (approximately 70%) and often remain asymptomatic until the fourth and fifth decades when patients may present with atrial arrhythmias (although exact timing and nature of presentation will be dependent upon the size of the shunt). Primum defects are usually detected earlier in life due to associated mitral and tricuspid valve defects. Sinus venosus defects are less common (approximately 10–15%) and occur in the upper septum where they may be associated with anomalous pulmonary drainage into the right atrium.

1.34   C: Regular clinical follow-up with repeat echocardiography

The assessment of the severity of mitral regurgitation and the timing of surgery can be extremely difficult. With the decline in rheumatic fever, prolapse is now the most common indication for mitral valve surgery in the UK. Ideally the valve should be repaired as opposed to replaced, if technically feasible, since this favours better preservation of post-operative left ventricular function and may negate the need for long-term anticoagulation if the patient is not in AF. Posterior leaflet prolapse is more common than anterior and is technically easier to repair. Indications for surgical intervention would include the development of symptoms, left ventricular dilatation or impairment (determined by sequential echo). However, in view of improved results with valve repair there is an increasing tendency to refer suitable patients with severe regurgitation for surgery at an earlier stage. This patient has preserved left ventricular function and moderate regurgitation and hence should undergo regular clinical and echocardiographical follow-up (eg three- to six-monthly). Written recommendations for SBE prophylaxis should be given to all patients with valvular disease. Warfarin (and possibly amiodarone) would be indicated if there is co-existent AF (including paroxysmal).

1.35   B: Bruce protocol exercise test

MI disqualifies HGV (group 2) licence holders from driving for six weeks. In order to fulfil DVLA requirements for HGV relicensing, Bruce protocol exercise testing should be performed. The patient will need to complete three stages of the Bruce protocol, off antianginal medication for 48 hours, and should remain free of angina, hypotension, sustained VT and/or significant ST-segment shift on ECG.

Clearly if symptoms continue or the exercise test is not satisfactory, angiography +/– percutaneous intervention would be required. Many centres perform angiography in particular young patients post-MI, although there is no direct evidence to support or contradict this approach. Whilst this may be considered, it is important to have objective knowledge of the patient's exercise tolerance/ symptomatic impairment to enable an appropriate management plan to be implemented.

Modified Bruce exercise testing is sometimes used as an early assessment post-MI prior to hospital discharge, or in patients unable to tolerate the formal Bruce protocol.

1.36   A: Intravenous β-blocker

Aortic dissection can be subdivided depending upon the site of origin of the dissection flap. Type A involves the ascending aorta (approximately 65%) and type B begins distal to the ascending aorta, usually just after the origin of the left subclavian artery. Management of these two presentations is very different. Type B dissections are generally treated medically, with aggressive control of blood pressure in an attempt to reduce complications. Surgical intervention is extremely difficult and carries a significant risk of paraplegia. This is therefore usually reserved for patients with complications such as aortic rupture, vital organ or limb ischaemia, or unremitting pain. However, endovascular repair is currently being tried in several specialised centres and this may provide a future alternative therapy. Early surgical intervention is indicated in the case of type A dissection and involves replacement of the diseased part of the aortic root and then re-establishing aortic continuity using a prosthetic graft. Precise blood pressure control is also mandatory in this setting.

In order to optimise blood pressure control an intravenous agent with a short half-life is preferred. Ideally, if not contraindicated, this would be in the form of a β-blocker such as propanolol or labetalol (α- and β-receptor blocker), which have beneficial effects on arterial wall stress by reducing arterial dP/dt (rate of change of arterial wall pressure). If β-blockers are contraindicated then appropriate intravenous alternatives would include nitroprusside or GTN. Oral agents can also be added and calcium-channel blockers reduce both arterial pressure and arterial dP/dt.

1.37   A: Dobutamine

This patient has an elevated PCWP, an impaired CI (cardiac output corrected for body surface area) and high SVR (evidence of peripheral vasoconstriction in an attempt to maintain blood pressure). Cardiogenic shock has developed as a result of extensive myocardial damage and hence inotropic support is required. Intravenous fluids should be avoided in view of the elevated PCWP (effectively left atrial pressure). Although IV GTN might be helpful in reducing pulmonary oedema (due to its vasodilatory effects), it would also adversely lower the systemic blood pressure in this case. Dobutamine, a β-receptor agonist, would be the optimum initial therapy since it is not only able to increase cardiac output (positive inotropic effects) but also results in a reduction in SVR (decrease in afterload). In contrast, noradrenaline, predominantly an α-receptor agonist, will result in further increases in SVR and therefore increases myocardial oxygen demand due to the increase in afterload. It is, however, the inotropic agent of choice for the management of septic shock where patients have marked vasodilatation. Dopamine (α-, β- and dopaminergic receptor agonist) is a relatively weak positive inotrope and at higher doses results in increased SVR. It is often used at low ('renal') dose in conjunction with other inotropes in an attempt to enhance renal perfusion (by renal vasodilatation) and subsequent diuresis, although direct evidence supporting a positive effect on survival is lacking.

1.38 E: Thrombolysis with tissue plasminogen activator

This patient has clinical features consistent with a haemodynamically compromising pulmonary embolus despite the initiation of LMWH therapy. Thrombolysis is indicated for patients with a proved pulmonary embolus who have evidence of haemodynamic compromise. Tissue plasminogen activator works faster than streptokinase and hence achieves re-perfusion more rapidly and is therefore the preferred choice in this setting. In patients with severe haemodynamic impairment, additional support with inotropes may also be required, together with cautious IV fluids (eg 500 ml). Whether thrombolysis is indicated in all patients with pulmonary emboli and right heart dilatation (usually diagnosed from echo) has yet to be confirmed.

Inferior vena cava filters are reserved for short-term use in patients with proved lower limb deep vein thrombosis (DVT) and evidence of pulmonary emboli, in whom anticoagulation is contraindicated.

1.39 C: *Staphylococcus epidermidis*

In the UK, *S. viridans* remain the commonest cause of native valve endocarditis. However, in the first year after valvular surgery the spectrum of infecting organisms is somewhat different, with coagulase-negative staphylococci being the most common (approximately 50%). When individual species are considered, the majority of these are *S. epidermidis*. It is presumed that these infections are nosocomial and, despite the delayed presentation, in many cases are derived from events occurring during the surgical admission. *S. aureus* is a virulent organism and systemic infections often run a fulminant course. Patients with SBE secondary to *S. aureus* are often exceedingly unwell with a relatively short history of illness. *Candida* infection is seen more commonly in intravenous drug abusers.

1.40 E: Pravastatin

The greatest evidence for the benefits for lipid-lowering in primary prevention comes from studies involving statins. Whilst benefit may also occur for other therapies without adverse effects, this is not entirely clear at present. Two major placebo-controlled statin studies have been performed, evaluating their role in primary prevention. WOSCOPS, using pravastatin, demonstrated a reduction in all-cause mortality of 22% and coronary heart disease incidence by 31% in men aged 45–64 years and an average cholesterol of 7 mmol/l at randomisation. The AFCAPS/TEXCAPS study evaluated the effect of lovastatin in healthy men and women with a mean cholesterol of 5.7 mmol/l and demonstrated a reduction in the incidence of major acute coronary heart disease events of 37%.

Current UK recommendations for primary prevention suggest treating elevated cholesterol with statins if annual coronary heart disease risk is above 3%. (Annual risk can be calculated from several published guidelines e.g. Sheffield tables.) Whilst the benefits of statins may well result from a 'class effect' it would seem appropriate to use one with proven results, if feasible.

1.41   B: Intravenous lidocaine (lignocaine)

The differential diagnosis of broad-complex tachycardia includes ventricular tachycardia (VT) or SVT with aberrant conduction. Whilst there are many ECG features which can help to differentiate between these two arrhythmias, if any doubt exists it should be treated as per VT. The presence of ischaemic heart disease or known impairment of ventricular function also significantly favours VT. Although this patient is currently haemodynamically stable it is important to treat the arrhythmia aggressively since decompensation can occur rapidly, particularly with a prior history of myocardial infarction. Although amiodarone would be an appropriate option, oral loading takes a long time to achieve therapeutic levels. Overdrive pacing is usually reserved for resistant cases of VT. Transoesophageal echo can be used to exclude left atrial thrombus prior to elective cardioversion but in the acute setting would be less likely to alter management and indeed if sedation is used may lead to haemodynamic embarrassment. If lidocaine proved ineffective then early DC cardioversion should be performed.

1.42   E: Increased ventricular rate

Cardiac output is the product of the heart rate and stroke volume. In turn, stroke volume is affected by pre-load, afterload and myocardial contractility. The degree of haemodynamic response depends upon the severity of exercise and the amount of muscle mass involved. Cardiac output can increase by as much as four to six times basal levels during strenuous exertion. Cardiac output and stroke volume are higher during supine rest when compared to the upright position. During exercise in the supine position the increase in cardiac output almost entirely results from an increase in heart rate.

During early exercise in the upright position enhanced cardiac output is achieved by increases in stroke volume (Frank–Starling mechanism) and heart rate. In contrast, during the later phases of exercise the increase in cardiac output is primarily due to increased heart rate. Strenuous exertion results in enhanced sympathetic discharge and withdrawal of parasympathetic stimulation, thereby promoting vasoconstriction; coronary, cerebral and skeletal muscle blood flow is, however, preserved. As exercise progresses, skeletal muscle blood flow increases further and total peripheral vascular resistance decreases.

1.43   C: Heavily calcified mitral valve

Percutaneous trans-septal mitral valvuloplasty can be extremely effective in treating symptomatic mitral stenosis. In addition, it may result in a decrease in previously elevated right heart pressures. Best results are seen in patients with pure mitral stenosis without valvular calcification, and in younger subjects where the subvalvular chordae have not become thickened and fused. Relative contra-indications to this approach include associated mitral regurgitation (which may be significantly increased by the procedure), a rigid, calcified valve and the presence of left atrial thrombus (usually visualised on TOE). Whilst atrial fibrillation and spontaneous contrast in the left atrium (seen on echo as 'swirling smoke' and thought to reflect sluggish blood flow) are associated with increased risk of left atrial thrombus formation, on their own they would not preclude intervention.

1.44   D: Reverse splitting of the second heart sound

Although the presence of LBBB on the resting ECG is commonly associated with significant underlying cardiac pathology, it may be a normal variant in a minority of cases. Causes of LBBB include: cardiomyopathy, ischaemic heart disease (including acute MI), hypertension, aortic valve disease and right ventricular pacing.

Clinical findings in subjects with LBBB will, to an extent, depend upon the exact nature of the underlying cardiac disease. For example, a displaced apex beat and third heart sound may be seen in dilated cardiomyopathy, whilst a fourth heart sound may be seen in cases of left ventricular hypertrophy or ischaemia. However, in all cases of LBBB there is early activation of the right side of the septum and the right ventricular myocardium. Trans-septal activation is transmyocardial and hence slowed. This means that left ventricular activation and subsequent contraction is delayed in comparison to the right ventricle, resulting in the clinical finding of reversed splitting of the second heart sound. In this fit, asymptomatic man this is therefore likely to be the most frequently found physical sign.

1.45   A: Acute rheumatic fever

Although the incidence of acute rheumatic fever has significantly declined in the western world, it is still a leading cause of cardiac morbidity in less industrialised countries. It occurs following infection with group A streptococcal species and it is thought that antigenic mimicry results in an autoimmune response and the subsequent clinical manifestations. The diagnosis is made clinically and generally involves the Jones criteria. In order to make the diagnosis there must be evidence of preceding streptococcal infection and either two major or one major and two minor criteria. In this case the patient has two major criteria – polyarthritis and evidence of carditis (most commonly involving the mitral valve, manifest as mitral incompetence). Other major criteria are chorea, erythema marginatum and subcutaneous nodules. This patient also has two minor criteria – fever and elevated inflammatory markers.

Although SBE is a significant possibility the history is usually more prolonged. The mean age of presentation for atrial myxoma is in the fifth decade, although they have been described in younger subjects. Kawasaki disease (mucocutaneous lymph node syndrome) is a generalised vasculitis of unknown aetiology, with 80% of cases occurring in children under five years. Cardiac findings include pancarditis and coronary artery abnormalities.

Systemic lupus erythematosus can have cardiac involvement (including pericarditis, myocarditis and, rarely, endocarditis) but the CRP is not normally elevated.

1.46   E: Warfarin

Although this patient has lone AF (no obvious aetiology and normal cardiac structure) it is important to continue formal anticoagulation with warfarin for a period of at least two to four weeks after successful cardioversion. Atrial mechanical stunning occurs post-cardioversion and lasts for several days and therefore patients remain at risk of thromboembolism even if atrial thrombi are excluded by pre-procedural TOE. Indeed, patients appear to be at particular risk when synchronised atrial contraction subsequently returns.

There is no evidence that digoxin helps to maintain sinus rhythm and indeed it may actually favour reversion to AF. Although amiodarone may help to maintain sinus rhythm there is no current consensus regarding its routine use in this setting.

1.47   B: Automated implantable cardiac defibrillator

Following failed sudden cardiac death, in the absence of a reversible cause (eg acute myocardial infarction), current recommendations (NICE guidelines) favour the insertion of an automated implantable cardiac defibrillator (AICD). This is also the intervention of choice for spontaneous, sustained VT causing syncope or significant haemodynamic compromise or sustained VT in the setting of impaired left ventricular function (ejection fraction < 35%).

If patients experience recurrent arrhythmias and hence frequent shocks then adjunctive therapy can be considered. This may include class III antiarrhythmics such as amiodarone and sotalol or electrophysiological studies and VT ablation.

1.48   B: Left internal mammary artery

The LAD supplies a major part of the left ventricular myocardium, including the anterior wall, apex and septum and as such it is important to choose the best option for revascularisation. The left internal mammary artery (LIMA) is usually free of atheroma and rarely develops intimal hyperplasia, unlike vein grafts. In contrast to the 40–60% patency seen in vein grafts at 10–12 years post-CABG, LIMA graft patency exceeds 90%. Patency for *in* situ LIMA grafts appears better than free grafts. Therefore the origin of the LIMA from the left subclavian artery is normally left intact, whilst the distal vessel is carefully mobilised and eventually anastomosed to the LAD (pedicle LIMA graft).

In younger patients full arterial revascularisation is becoming increasingly attempted with additional use of RIMA anastomosis to the right coronary artery and harvesting of radial arteries.

1.49   B: Hypertrophic cardiomyopathy

The classic finding in hypertrophic cardiomyopathy (HCM) is inappropriate hypertrophy of the myocardium without an obvious cause. The ventricular cavity is usually small and microscopic examination reveals gross disorganisation of muscle bundles and myofibrillar disarray. Familial HCM is inherited in an autosomal dominant manner, accounting for approximately 50% of cases. It is thought that many of the sporadic cases result from spontaneous mutations. Although many patients are asymptomatic and identified by screening, symptoms include dyspnoea, classic angina, palpitations and dizziness. The majority of symptoms are exacerbated with exercise. Unfortunately, in some the first presentation is with sudden death. Syncope may result from inadequate cardiac output during exercise or arrhythmias.

The resting ECG is usually abnormal and the commonest features include ST-segment and T-wave abnormalities, LVH with the tallest complexes in the mid-precordial leads and prominent Q waves (inferior and precordial).

Supravalvular aortic stenosis is seen in several different clinical settings, for example as a sporadic, isolated congenital lesion or as part of a clinical syndrome eg Williams' syndrome (elfin facies, mental impairment, hypercalcaemia and peripheral pulmonary stenoses).

1.50   B: Endocardial cushion defect

The most common causes of morbidity and mortality in Down's syndrome are congenital heart defects, which are present in 40–50% of cases. The most characteristic cardiac abnormality is a defect of endocardial cushion closure. This results from varying degrees of incomplete development of the inferior portion of the atrial septum, the inflow portion of the ventricular septum and the atrioventricular valves. Therefore abnormalities may range from a small ostium primum ASD to an extensive defect that also involves the ventricular septum, together with the mitral and tricuspid valves.

Patients with trisomy 21 seem to have a particular propensity to develop pulmonary hypertension in situations resulting in increased pulmonary blood flow, irrespective of the complexity of the underlying defect. Aortic and pulmonary valve cusps are predisposed to develop fenestrations in adulthood, resulting in valvular incompetence. Mitral valve prolapse is also found with increased frequency in Down's syndrome.

2.1   D: He is likely to have had a splenectomy at the time of laparotomy for peptic ulceration

This is an adult patient who has had a splenectomy performed as an 'encore' during a gastrectomy operation in the days before H_2-antagonists and proton pump inhibitors, when the requirements for post-splenectomy infection prophylaxis were less clear than they are now. The post-splenectomy blood film shows Howell–Jolly bodies (nuclear remnants within the red cells which would normally be removed by the pitting function of the spleen) and occasional target cells and spherocytes, which are imperfect red cells that are normally removed from the circulation by a functioning spleen. After a splenectomy patients may also demonstrate an enhanced neutrophil and platelet response to inflammation and may have a thrombocytosis. He would be advised to have lifelong penicillin V prophylaxis, *Haemophilus influenzae* and meningococcal C immunisation. A warning card and information pamphlet is available. Pneumococcal immunisation at this stage may be associated with increased risk of reaction and should probably be delayed until the following winter. Antibiotics most suitable for a community-acquired lobar pneumonia would be amoxicillin plus clarithromycin, though many other choices would be suitable.

2.2   D: Bone marrow aspirate

The blood count is typical of myelodysplasia (MDS), confirmed by the finding of hypo-granular neutrophils and neutrophils that have only one or two lobes to their nucleus. Pelger–Huët anomaly is a benign inherited condition associated with failure of segmentation of neutrophil nuclei. Pseudo-Pelger morphology is one of the dysplastic changes found in the blood in myelodysplasia. A monocytosis is also a very frequent finding in MDS, most notably in chronic myelomonocytic leukaemia. Although B_{12} and folate deficiency result in a macrocytic anaemia, the severity of thrombocytopenia and neutropenia in this case makes this unlikely to be the cause of the anaemia, though of course these vitamin levels should be checked as routine. Iron deficiency produces a microcytic anaemia; an elevated ferritin may be found in the 'refractory anaemia with ring sideroblast' variety of MDS (also known as primary sideroblastic anaemia). Bone marrow aspirate would be likely to show a collection of dysplastic changes such as nuclear fragmentation, intercytoplasmic bridging of erythroblasts and megaloblastoid change. Although an elevated haemoglobin F may be found in the myelodysplastic states, and very rarely an acquired haemoglobin H, screening for haemoglobinopathies is unlikely to prove rewarding. Reticulocytes are large red cells and a high reticulocyte count may produce a macrocytosis. However one would expect a film comment of 'polychromasia' and it would be difficult to tie this in with the thrombocytopenia and neutropenia.

2.3   E: Induction chemotherapy would usually consist of cytosine and an anthracycline

Young patients with acute myeloid leukaemia (AML) are treated with conventional chemotherapy if the prognosis appears good, and bone marrow transplant (associated with a higher treatment-related mortality) if the prognosis appears poor with conventional treatment. Cytogenetic abnormality and response to the first course of chemotherapy determine prognosis in AML. Three cytogenetic abnormalities that are associated with a good prognosis are: t(8;21) – commonest in the FAB morphological type M2; t(15;17) – found in acute promyelocytic leukaemia; and inversion 16 – found in acute myelomonocytic leukaemia with increased eosinophils. Three cytogenetic abnormalities that are associated with a particularly poor prognosis and recommendation to bone marrow allograft are: t(9;22) – the truncated chromosome 22 being Philadelphia chromosome; and deletion of all or part of chromosomes 5 or 7. Failure to go into remission after the first course of treatment is also bad news. Vincristine and steroids are the principal remission-inducing drugs for acute lymphoblastic leukaemia, whereas cytosine and an anthracycline will almost always feature in an AML induction regimen. A high-risk matched unrelated donor transplant is not justified in this young woman with good-prognosis cytogenetics unless she fails to go into remission with the first course of chemotherapy.

2.4   A: The clinical and pathological features may all be related to the post-ictal state

This lady has a history typical of thrombotic thrombocytopenic purpura (TTP). An excess of high molecular weight von Willebrand's factor sticks platelets to the inside of her vascular endothelium, resulting in their activation and local triggering of the coagulation cascade. Fibrin formation in small blood vessels chops up passing red cells, resulting in anaemia and reticulocytosis. Some of these red cells can re-seal themselves, continuing as half red cells (helmet cells) or, if subject to multiple fibrin collisions, as fragmented cells. Such a micro-angiopathic blood picture may be found in other conditions such as disseminated intravascular coagulation, but in this condition abnormality of the coagulation screening tests would be expected. Infection with *E. coli* O157 may precipitate haemolytic uraemic syndrome, in which renal failure is a major feature as opposed to neurological problems as in TTP.

2.5   B: Stainable bone marrow iron

There is a high probability of iron deficiency due to menorrhagia and a diet with inadequate red meat, which is the richest source of dietary iron. Serum ferritin is reduced in iron deficiency and increased in iron overload and provides a useful guide to body iron stores. However, it may be falsely elevated into the normal range in patients who have an inflammatory condition as ferritin is an acute phase reactant, similar to CRP, immunoglobulins and fibrinogen. In iron deficiency there will be no stainable iron in the bone marrow though this investigation is too invasive to perform in the diagnosis of most cases! It is possible to have a normal haemoglobin level but no stainable iron stores if iron from broken-down red cells is efficiently reprocessed into haemoglobin. In iron deficiency the serum iron is low and the total iron-binding capacity (TIBC – equivalent to transferrin) is raised. Dividing one by the other gives a reduced transferrin saturation in iron deficiency. Measurement of zinc protoporphyrin is used as a screening test for iron deficiency, when it is elevated. In β-thalassaemia trait, which would be in the differential diagnosis of this girl's microcytic anaemia, an elevated haemoglobin A_2 level is a common finding. Inability to make the β-globin chains of haemoglobin A results in compensation by making more haemoglobin A_2 which does not need   β-globin chains, having instead δ-globin chains.

2.6   E: Diastolic murmur at the cardiac apex

In β-thalassaemia major virtually no β chains can be manufactured and consequently progressive anaemia results during the attempted physiological switch from Hb F to Hb A during the first year of life. Nucleated red cells are a consistent feature of the blood film in β-thalassaemia major and help to differentiate this condition from other causes of severe microcytic anaemia, such as iron deficiency. In the un-transfused patient skeletal changes such as pushing forward of the mandible and maxilla (prognathism), bossing of skull, and stunting of growth may be found. These skeletal changes are secondary to the severe erythroid hyperplasia, most of which is ineffective in maintaining a normal haemoglobin level. Regular blood transfusions are required as well as a chelating agent such as desferrioxamine in order to prevent iron overload that results in cardiomyopathy, endocrinopathy and cirrhosis.

An ejection systolic murmur may be heard in any severe form of anaemia due to increased blood flow through the heart, but not a diastolic murmur.

2.7   A: It is the optimal replacement fluid following major burns

Fresh frozen plasma is commonly used for the replacement of multiple coagulation factor deficiencies such as those in disseminated intravascular coagulation, warfarin overdose with haemorrhage, and after massive transfusion. FFP contains blood group antibodies and therefore the patient's blood group should be known. If not, group AB fresh frozen plasma does contain anti-A or anti-B antibodies so can be given to recipients of any ABO blood group. In severe burns the most appropriate fluid for volume replacement is albumin, as large amounts of this weep from the denuded body surfaces. Albumin is heat-treated to inactivate viruses, and does not contain blood group antibodies.

2.8   C: Repeat coagulation screen on fresh sample

A prolonged thrombin time in isolation, in this clinical situation, is most likely to have resulted from heparin contamination of the blood sample used for the coagulation screen. It is likely to have been drawn from an indwelling catheter with insufficient removal of heparin-contaminated blood. A repeat coagulation screen on a fresh sample is likely to be normal. The thrombin time is not used for dose control of conventional heparin because it is so sensitive to heparin effect, the APTT being a better substitute. Sometimes it is possible for the laboratory to neutralise the heparin in the sample with protamine to demonstrate that the prolonged thrombin time is an artefact due to heparin contamination. Prolongation of the thrombin time may be seen in heparin, disseminated intravascular coagulation (DIC), and in the presence of a low fibrinogen. Measurement of FDPs is a reasonable option in DIC but these may be elevated in a trauma case.

2.9   B: Coagulation screen

This woman has a deep venous thrombosis and probable pulmonary embolus in the puerperal period. There is a clear clinical reason for the thrombosis and in the absence of a personal or family history of thrombosis, screening for thrombophilia is not indicated. There is no reason to measure clotting factor IX. A coagulation screen may reasonably be performed before starting patients on anticoagulant therapy as a baseline.

2.10   D: Continue heparin infusion at current rate

The aim of conventional heparin therapy, which should be given by continuous infusion in order to maintain constant blood levels, is to prolong the APTT by 1.5–2.5 times the control value. This woman is therefore adequately anticoagulated and she may continue conventional heparin treatment. The equivalence of low molecular weight heparin in the treatment of pulmonary embolism has been shown but it has not been demonstrated to be superior and is considerably more expensive. Warfarin treatment takes 72 hours to take full effect; therefore heparin treatment will need to be continued until the INR (measuring warfarin effect) exceeds 2.0.

2.11   C: Idiopathic cold haemagglutinin disease

In this lady with anaemia and cold agglutinins the most likely cause is idiopathic cold haemagglutinin disease (CHAD). Chronic B cell lymphoproliferative disorders such as CLL may be associated with cold agglutinins, but she has no lymphocytosis and therefore is unlikely to have CLL. A *Mycoplasma* chest infection would be likely to have been clinically evident. Glandular fever tends to be a disease of the teenage years and would be exceptional in this elderly lady. All of the answers may be associated with cold agglutinins with the exception of tertiary syphilis, which historically is associated with paroxysmal cold haemo-globinuria (PCH – due to an IgG non-agglutinating antibody that causes intravascular haemolysis and haemoglobinuria by the action of complement). PCH is most commonly seen nowadays in children with viral infections.

2.12   E: Balanced expression of kappa and lambda light chain expression of surface immunoglobulin on blood lymphocytes

More than 95% of cases of chronic lymphocytic leukaemia are of B cell lineage. Curiously they almost always express a T cell antigen CD5, as well as the usual B cell antigens such as CD19. B cells are responsible for immunoglobulin production and there may be deranged antibody production, with low immunoglobulin levels associated with predisposition to infection and auto-immune phenomenon of which the commonest is a positive direct antiglobulin test, sometimes associated with warm autoimmune haemolytic anaemia. Establishment of clonality is important in the diagnosis of neoplasia and one would expect these lymphocytes to either all express kappa light chains or all express lambda. Balanced production would be more in keeping with a reactive lymphocytosis, but if the other investigations suggest CLL this test should probably be repeated.

2.13   D: Multiple myeloma

It is quite reasonable to investigate this girl for any of the first three causes of macrocytosis. Folate deficiency may be caused by antiepileptic medication and it is controversial whether the fits get worse if the folate deficiency is corrected. Liver disease causes macrocytosis by interfering with the construction of the lipid bilayer of the red cell membrane. The occurrence of multiple myeloma would be exceptional in a girl of this age group, though macrocytosis is found in patients with multiple myeloma. There is no particular reason why she should have autoimmune haemolytic anaemia and this is fairly low down the list of diagnostic possibilities.

2.14   A: The action of antithrombin on fibrinogen results in the development of a fibrin clot

In the terminal events of the coagulation cascade, prothrombin is converted to thrombin and thrombin acts on fibrinogen, converting it to fibrin clot. Blood contains the coagulation factors which generally clot, and natural anticoagulants that inhibit this process. These include protein C, protein S (which are vitamin K-dependent anticoagulants) and antithrombin (previously called antithrombin III). The prothrombin time is prolonged by deficiency of factors within the extrinsic and final coagulation pathways, that is, factors VII, X, V and prothrombin. The APTT is prolonged by deficiencies within the intrinsic coagulation pathway and final common pathway, that is, factors XII, XI, VIII, IX, V and prothrombin. Only deficiency of fibrinogen, or some inhibitor of the conversion of fibrinogen to fibrin clot such as heparin, or high levels of FDPs prolong the thrombin time.

2.15   C: Factor VIII inhibitor screen

The most likely cause of his persistent haemarthrosis is the development of antibodies against factor VIII, although many haemophiliacs do develop a 'target joint' subject to recurrent haemarthrosis due to synovial hyperplasia and secondary joint damage. This is a difficult situation to treat. The most relevant investigation to detect these would be a screen for factor VIII inhibitor antibodies. He is unlikely to have developed gout. Joint aspiration is rarely performed in haemophilia, effective correction of the coagulation abnormality being the best treatment.

2.16　E: Patient immunisation against influenza A pre-transplant

Post-transplant pneumonitis is a difficult problem that may be due to a variety of infective causes. Cytomegalovirus infection suggests a strong possibility that the donor or recipient are CMV antibody-positive, implying that they have CMV resident in their lymphocytes. This may proliferate and cause severe infection during periods of immunosuppression. If donor and recipient are CMV-negative then blood products for these patients should be derived from CMV-negative blood donors. It is usual to monitor the CMV viral load in the post-transplant period so pre-emptive treatment with ganciclovir or foscarnet can be commenced as soon as there is evidence of CMV viral replication.

Prophylaxis against *Pneumocystis carinii* can be effectively given by low doses of oral co-trimoxazole though it is usual to use monthly nebulised pentamidine if the blood counts are precarious as co-trimoxazole can suppress haematopoiesis. Itraconazole is an oral antifungal agent with some activity against *Aspergillus* though it is more usual to have lumpy chest disease rather than the diffuse ground-glass shadowing if fungus were its cause. Radiotherapy may result in a post-transplant aseptic pneumonitis, effectively treated by steroids, but this is relatively rare with good lung shielding and is usually seen earlier in the course of transplantation. Any benefits of immunisation prior to the transplant procedure would be best seen by immunising the donor, whose immune system is implanted into the recipient.

2.17　E: Measurement of CD55 and CD59 surface antigen on peripheral blood leukocytes and platelets

The history is typical of paroxysmal nocturnal haemoglobinuria (PNH). In this rare disorder there is complement-mediated lysis of red cells, white cells and platelets, resulting in a pancytopenia. Sometimes haematopoietic stem cells are also affected, giving rise to aplastic anaemia. Intravascular lysis of red cells results in haemoglobinuria and the release of tissue factor from lysed cells gives an acquired thrombophilia, so that patients may present with thrombotic problems which are a common cause of death in this disease. The disease is due to the lack of a transmembrane glycoprotein that acts as an anchor for various molecules, including complement activators and CD antigens. Although Ham's test is usually positive in PNH, in this case the patient has been transfused with normal red cells so this may result in a negative result as red cells are used for this test. The membrane defect can however be revealed by measurement of antigens such as CD55 and CD59 on other blood cells. Urinary haemosiderin merely tells us that the patient has had chronic haemoglobinuria, some of the haemoglobin being internalised within tubular cells which are later shed into the urinary deposit and give a positive stain for iron. The Donath–Landsteiner test detects the complement-dependent, cold-acting antibody found in paroxysmal cold haemoglobinuria, a different disease.

2.18   C: It is free of risk of hepatitis transmission

Cryoprecipitate is prepared by thawing fresh frozen plasma, when curd-like precipitate forms at the bottom of the bag that may be harvested and is particularly rich in fibrinogen factor VII and von Willebrand's factor. Because heat-detergent inactivates concentrates of factor VII and von Willebrand's factor these are preferred for the treatment of von Willebrand's disease rather than cryoprecipitate, which has not gone through a viral inactivation stage and therefore may carry a very small risk of hepatitis transmission. Cryoprecipitate is most commonly used for the correction of a low fibrinogen in patients with disseminated intravascular coagulation or massive transfusion. The von Willebrand's factor in the cryoprecipitate can ameliorate bleeding in uraemic patients but DDAVP administration causes endothelial cells to secrete stored von Willebrand's factor and may be a more suitable treatment of uraemic platelet defect.

2.19   D: G-CSF carries no risk of viral transmission

G-CSF is a recombinant protein and therefore there is no risk of viral disease transmission. G-CSF stimulates committed myeloid progenitor cells and is therefore of most use when the primitive stem cells have differentiated into the early myeloid lineage. It may shorten periods of post-chemotherapy neutropenia by a few days. It is best given after chemotherapy rather than immediately before as it may stimulate granulocyte precursors into division, making them more susceptible to the suppressive effects of cytotoxic chemotherapy. Most modern trials have shown the benefits of accelerated chemotherapy rather than increasing the interval between courses to allow full count recovery.

2.20   B: Recent febrile illness associated with high titres against parvovirus B19

Chemotherapy and radiotherapy are the most common causes of a hypoplastic marrow with pancytopenia. Busulfan is an old-fashioned cytotoxic treatment for CML, but is still used and the possibility of deliberate poisoning should always be considered. An idiosyncratic reaction to drugs may result in aplastic anaemia; phenylbutazone and chloramphenicol are well-known examples. If in doubt the drug should be stopped or changed. A severe aplastic anaemia can follow any viral hepatitis, often after recovery of the liver function tests. PNH has an association with aplastic anaemia, as the haematopoietic stem cells are more liable to complement lysis, like the cells in the peripheral blood. Parvovirus B19 causes pure red cell aplasia, not aplastic anaemia. It infects the erythroblasts in the bone marrow, shutting down red cell production for a few days. In normal people, whose red cells have a three-month lifespan, stopping red cell production for a few days is of no consequence, but in patients with chronic congenital haemolytic anaemia a severe anaemia may result in aplastic crisis. However the white cell and platelet counts remain normal and this is not true of aplastic anaemia.

2.21 C: The patient is unusually sensitive to the effect of warfarin

The heparin dose should be adjusted to obtain an APTT ratio of 1.5 to 2.5. This patient is correctly heparinised. Over-heparinisation can cause prolongation of the INR, which normally reflects warfarin effect. Achieving an INR of 1.8 only 12 hours after the first dose indicates increased warfarin sensitivity or abnormal liver function tests at the start of therapy; normally the effects of warfarin are not seen for 48–72 hours after starting treatment. The therapeutic INR range for DVT/PE and AF is 2–3; for recurrent thrombosis on warfarin or artificial heart valves the range is 3–4.5. The INR is the prothrombin ratio raised to the power of the sensitivity index of the thromboplastin used in the test. In simpler terms it is the prothrombin ratio multiplied by a 'fiddle factor' to bring it in line with the results of other laboratories, so that the INR should be the same in any laboratory performing the test.

2.22 E: Elevated TSH and low free thyroxine

β-thalassaemia trait results in a microcytic hypochromic anaemia difficult to differentiate from iron deficiency except that the haemoglobin is usually over 9 g/dl. Consequently this lady is much more likely to have iron deficiency. In pernicious anaemia lack of gastric acid prevents iron being split from protein to allow its absorption, so patients with this disease frequently suffer iron deficiency. Non-steroidal anti-inflammatory drug (NSAID) treatment may cause gastric erosions and impair platelet function, enhancing chronic GI bleeding which may result in iron deficiency. The most easily absorbed form of iron in the diet is in red meat and vegetarians have a more precarious iron status than meat eaters. The anaemia of hypothyroidism is usually macrocytic rather than microcytic.

2.23 D: Anorexia and malaise

Increase in haemoglobin level results in an increased whole blood viscosity that may exacerbate hypertension already present in patients with renal failure. Increased blood viscosity may also predispose to a higher incidence of thrombosis and it is usual to limit the haemoglobin level to around 10 g/dl in renal patients. Improvement in haemoglobin level often results in a greater feeling of wellbeing and improved appetite. Pure red cell aplasia is a very rare unwanted effect of erythropoietin administration due to the stimulation of antibodies by administered EPO that cross-reacts with the patient's endogenous erythropoietin. A similar problem has been reported in trials of human recombinant thrombopoietin.

2.24 B: Haemoglobin electrophoresis

This man has leukoerythroblastic anaemia: nucleated red cells and primitive white cells in the peripheral blood. Unless the patient is seriously ill this is likely to be due to bone marrow infiltration. Investigations should include a search for primary tumours that characteristically metastasise to bone (lung, thyroid, kidney, breast, prostate) as well as haematological malignancies such as myeloma.

2.25 C: The ABO type of individuals can change during some illnesses, eg acute myeloid leukaemia

Naturally occurring anti-A and anti-B antibodies are IgM (agglutinating and non-placenta-passing). IgG antibodies may be made in response to immunological stimulation by incompatible red cells such as those transmitted from fetus to mother during pregnancy. These IgG anti-A or anti-B antibodies may cause ABO haemolytic disease of the newborn. Changing of an ABO blood group is an exceptional event but may be found after bone marrow transplantation, in some cases of acute myeloid leukaemia affecting the erythroid lineage, and in some cases of enteric disease when the red cells of non-group B individuals may acquire a B antigen. Group O is the commonest blood group in all races. Persons who are group O are universal donors for red cells but persons of blood group AB are universal donors for fresh frozen plasma as their plasma contains neither anti-A nor anti-B.

2.26 E: Barium enema

Investigations need to establish if there is significant haemolysis occurring and if there is an associated autoimmune disorder. Rarely, autoimmune haemolytic anaemia is associated with low-grade lymphoproliferative disorders. Drugs associated with a Coombs'-positive haemolytic anaemia are mefenamic acid, α-methyldopa, and high-dose penicillin.

2.27 A: Stop heparin and commence heparinoid

The history is strongly suggestive of heparin-induced thrombocytopenia (HIT). This condition is associated with immunological activation of platelets and an increased risk of further thrombosis. Anticoagulation should not be stopped. HIT may be seen with low molecular weight heparin so this is not a suitable alternative. Either a heparinoid such as danaparoid or recombinant hirudin should be used, after taking haematological advice.

2.28 D: Measurement of serum levels after oral therapy provides a good guide to the efficacy of treatment

Parenteral B_{12} treatment is only required quarterly, assuming that hydroxocobalamin at a dose of 1 mg is given intramuscularly. This is derived from bacterial fermentation so can be used in vegans. Oral therapy would be reasonable here if the dietary history is clear. After oral replacement therapy serum levels should be checked to ensure they have normalised and the blood count checked to ensure resolution of the macrocytic anaemia. When the cause of a macrocytic anaemia is uncertain both B_{12} and folic acid should be administered until the blood levels are available as folic acid on its own may exacerbate neurological damage in B_{12} deficiency.

2.29 E: Thrombotic thrombocytopenic purpura

Thrombotic thrombocytopenic purpura is a disorder characterised by severe thrombocytopenia, purpura, fragmentation haemolysis and ischaemic organ damage to the brain and kidney. Extensive deposition of arterial thrombi occurs. An immune-mediated mechanism involving the production of an antibody which inhibits von Willebrand's factor (cleaving protease) has been described. Plasma exchange and plasma infusions are the most effective therapy. Aspirin, corticosteroids and other agents, such as vincristine, azathioprine and cyclophosphamide may be of benefit. Haemolytic uraemic syndrome in children is a similar disorder but damage is confined to the kidney.

2.30 A: Major ABO incompatibility

Haemolytic transfusion reactions can be immediate or delayed. Immediate life-threatening reactions with massive intravascular haemolysis are caused by complement-activating IgG or IgM antibodies. These are usually ABO antibodies and the severity depends on the recipient's titre of antibody. Reactions can occur after the transfusion of only a few millilitres of blood. Immediate clinical features include back pain, flushing, headache, shortness of breath, vomiting, rigors, urticaria, pyrexia, tachycardia and hypotension. Many of these features will be masked in the anaesthetised patient. Evidence of red cell destruction with haemoglobinuria and disseminated intravascular coagulation can occur. In the UK all such incidents are reported through the SHOT (serious hazards of transfusion) system and they should be investigated locally.

2.31   D: Hereditary spherocytosis

Hereditary spherocytosis is the commonest hereditary haemolytic anaemia in Northern Europeans. Inheritance is usually autosomal dominant but can be autosomal recessive. It is due to a defect in the structural proteins of the red cell membrane, including ankyrin, anion exchanger, protein 4.2 and spectrin. The patients present with anaemia, fluctuating jaundice, splenomegaly and pigment gallstones. The degree of anaemia tends to be the same in families. The blood film shows microspherocytes. Patients' red cells show increased haemolysis compared to normal in the osmotic fragility test. The mainstay of treatment is splenectomy in those who have sufficient haemolysis to justify this, or gallstones.

2.32   B: Chronic myeloid leukaemia

Chronic myeloid leukaemia is an acquired clonal proliferative disorder. In most cases there is a reciprocal translocation between the long arms of chromosomes 9 and 22 resulting in an abnormal chromosome 22 (the Philadelphia chromosome) and the formation of a new fusion gene, *bcr/abl*. Clinically, the patients are often middle-aged but can present in any age group. Symptoms are related to anaemia and the raised white cell count. There is usually splenomegaly which may be symptomatic. The white cell count is raised up to $500 \times 10^9/l$ with a complete spectrum of cells in the peripheral blood, anaemia, and often a raised platelet count. Agents like hydroxyurea and busulfan control the white cell count. Allogeneic bone marrow transplant offers the chance of cure in suitable candidates. The new tyrosine kinase inhibitor, STI 571 (Glivec) may be an important agent in the treatment of the disease. The natural course of the disease involves transformation to acute leukaemia in a median period of three to four years.

2.33   C: Multiple myeloma

Multiple myeloma is characterised by a neoplastic monoclonal proliferation of plasma cells in the bone marrow. Clinical features include bone pain and pathological fractures, anaemia, recurrent infections, abnormal bleeding tendency, renal failure and hyperviscosity syndrome. It is diagnosed by finding two out of three of: 1) a paraprotein band in the serum or urine or both; 2) increased and often abnormal plasma cells in the bone marrow; and 3) lytic lesions on skeletal survey. Treatment involves resuscitation, treatment of renal failure, pain relief and, in older patients, melphalan and prednisolone. In younger patients more intensive combination chemotherapy regimens and a bone marrow transplant procedure may be considered.

2.34   B: Vitamin B$_{12}$, folic acid and iron supplements and slow transfusion of 1–2 units of packed cells if clinically indicated

Addisonian pernicious anaemia due to vitamin B$_{12}$ deficiency is usually caused by atrophy of the stomach, which is probably autoimmune in origin. It is more common in women than in men and the peak incidence is in older age groups. Patients present insidiously with gradual onset of symptoms and signs of anaemia and mild jaundice due to increased haemoglobin breakdown. Treatment with vitamin B$_{12}$ and folic acid is usually given until the exact vitamin deficiency is determined and also oral iron as requirements can increase when red cell production commences. Potassium levels should be monitored and potassium replacement may be required. Heart failure should be corrected. Blood transfusion should be avoided as it may cause circulatory overload. If judged to be essential because of anoxia, however, 1–2 units should be given slowly with the possibility of exchange transfusion being considered.

2.35   C: G6PD deficiency

Glucose-6-phosphate dehydrogenase oxidises glucose-6-phosphate (G6P) to 6-phosphogluconolactone (6PG) with concomitant reduction of nicotinamide adenine dinucleotide phosphate (NADP) to the reduced form NADPH. G6PD is essential to protect red cells from oxidative damage. The gene is located on the long arm of the X chromosome (Xq28). The deficiency affects over 400 million people worldwide. In most cases it exists as a balanced polymorphism, affected individuals having the advantage of resistance to malaria. Most people are asymptomatic unless exposed to an oxidising agent but a small subset of cases have chronic haemolysis. On exposure to infection or drugs or on ingestion of fava beans, patients rapidly develop intravascular haemolysis with haemoglobinuria. The blood film shows 'bite' cells and 'blister' cells which have had Heinz bodies (oxidised denatured haemoglobin) removed by the spleen. Treatment consists of stopping the offending drug, maintaining a high urine output and transfusing if necessary.

2.36   C: Clozapine

The lower limit of the neutrophil count is 2.5 x 10^9/l except in blacks or those from the Middle East where 1.5 x 10^9/l is acceptable. Recurrent infections are likely to occur when the neutrophil count falls below 0.5 x 10^9/l. Selective neutropenia due to individual susceptibility to an agent may follow a large number of different drugs. The mechanism of the neutropenia may be direct toxic damage to a bone marrow precursor cell or may stimulate an immune mechanism which damages neutophils or their precursors. A drug-hapten mechanism may be responsible in some cases. Drugs which can induce neutropenia   include antibacterials, anticonvulsants, anti-inflammatory drugs, antithyroids, hypoglycaemics, pheno-thiazines, psychotropics and antidepressants and other agents such as gold and penicillamine. Clozapine is an antipsychotic drug used in the treatment of schizophrenia in patients unresponsive to, or intolerant of, conventional antipsychotic agents.

2.37   B: Graft-versus-host disease

Graft-versus-host disease is caused by donor-derived immune cells, particularly T cells, reacting against the recipient. The incidence increases with age. If it occurs before 100 days it is described as acute and after that as chronic. Acute graft-versus-host disease involves the skin, gut and liver. The skin rash typically involves the palms of the hands and soles of the feet but may involve the whole body. The diagnosis is confirmed by biopsy. The gut manifestations are diarrhoea and vomiting. Typically the liver enzymes show elevation of the bilirubin and ALP with relatively normal levels of the other enzymes. Chronic graft-versus-host disease typically follows from the acute form and involves the skin, oral mucosa and other lacrimal glands, and the joints and other serosal surfaces. The problem is prevented by immune suppression, including ciclosporin, methotrexate, cortico-steroids and T cell depletion. Should it be manifest, then treatment is with corticosteroids or antilymphocyte globulin (ALG).

2.38   D: Haemochromatosis

Hereditary haemochromatosis is an autosomal recessive disorder of iron metabolism resulting in excess intestinal absorption and cellular deposition of iron which is relatively common in people of Northern European origin. The disease was found to be associated with the HLA-A3 allele and now in over 83% of patients the *HFE* gene, located on chromosome 6, has been discovered to be mutated. The disorder presents with non-specific complaints such as malaise, fatigue, arthralgia, sexual dysfunction and abdominal pain. The classical 'bronze diabetes' with hepatic fibrosis and cirrhosis, cardiomyopathy, endocrine dysfunction and liver cancer presents after prolonged iron overloading when the diagnosis is made late. Transferrin saturation (serum iron/total iron binding capacity) is the most sensitive biochemical marker of iron overload. A transferrin saturation of > 55% in males or > 50% in females merits investigation for haemochromatosis. Treatment is with venesection. It is recommended that weekly phlebotomy is carried out until the serum ferritin is 10–20 µg/l and then maintenance phlebotomy three or four times a year to maintain the serum ferritin at 50 µg/l. Liver biopsy should be considered with a serum ferritin of greater than 400 µg/l in men and 200 µg/l in women to determine the amount of stainable iron and assess for injury.

2.39   E: Sideroblastic anaemia

In sideroblastic anaemia there are hypochromic red cells in the peripheral blood (suggesting iron deficiency) but increased bone marrow iron. Erythroblasts contain abnormal iron granules, characteristically in the mitochondria positioned round the nucleus, hence they are known as ring sideroblasts. There is a defect of haem synthesis. It is classified into hereditary and acquired forms. The hereditary form may be due to δ-aminolevulinate synthase-2 deficiency. Acquired forms include myelodysplasia, drugs, including antituberculous medication, and alcohol. Some patients may respond to pyridoxine and folic acid but blood transfusion may be the only way to maintain the haemoglobin.

2.40   A: Immediate exchange transfusion

Sickle cell anaemia may remain undiagnosed until adult life and a crisis can be precipitated by a move to a colder climate. Prophylactic treatment includes avoidance of factors likely to cause crisis, good general nutrition, folic acid, pneumococcal vaccination and oral penicillin. Crises are treated with rehydration, antibiotics if infection is a factor, and strong analgesics. Exchange transfusion is indicated if there is neurological damage, visceral sequestration crises or recurrent painful crises. Achieving a Hb S level of less than 30% may limit the neurological damage. There may be problems in obtaining compatible blood for transfusion.

2.41   E: α-Thalassaemia major

α-Thalassaemia is usually due to deletions of the alpha–globin gene. There are two α-globin genes on each chromosome 16. All four genes must be deleted for α-thalassaemia major to occur. In some populations with α-thalassaemia trait one α-globin gene is missing on each chromosome 16 and thus full-blown α-thalassaemia will not occur in offspring of affected parents. However, in other ethnic groups such as Chinese populations, individuals with α-thalassaemia trait tend to have two missing α-globin genes on the same chromosome 16 and thus if both parents have the trait there is a one in four chance that the fetus will have α-thalassaemia major which leads to failure of fetal haemoglobin production and death in utero from hydrops fetalis.

2.42   B: Aplastic anaemia

Aplastic anaemia is pancytopenia resulting from failure of the bone marrow. It can be congenital (eg Fanconi's anaemia) or acquired. The acquired form can be idiopathic or secondary to ionising radiation, chemicals, drugs or infections (eg viral hepatitis). The result is a reduction in the number of pluripotential stem cells, either due to their destruction or an immune reaction against them. The peak incidence of the acquired form is 30 years and the patients present with symptoms and signs of anaemia, neutropenia and thrombocytopenia. Treatment initially involves removal of the cause and supportive treatment. Specific treatment includes immune suppression with antilymphocyte globulin, ciclosporin and methylprednisolone. Bone marrow transplantation may be curative if a suitable donor is available. Androgens and haematopoietic growth factors may also have a role to play.

2.43   C: Heparin-induced thrombocytopenia

Type I heparin-induced thrombocytopenia occurs within a few days of starting heparin: the platelet count rarely falls below 100 x 10^9/l and does not usually cause a clinical problem. Type II heparin-induced thrombocytopenia arises as a haemato-immunological adverse reaction after 5–15 days of heparin and is associated with thrombosis. It arises because of a reaction between heparin, platelet factor 4 and immunoglobulin binding to a specific receptor on the platelet surface. The complex is then phagocytosed and thrombosis arises either from direct platelet activation or immune injury to endothelium with tissue factor activation and subsequent activation of the coagulation cascade. Specific laboratory tests including an ELISA and flow cytometry are available. Treatment involves stopping all heparin immediately. No platelets should be given despite the low platelet count and alternative anticoagulation such as hirudin, danaparoid sodium or thrombolysis should be used.

2.44   E: von Willebrand's disease

von Willebrand's disease is a disorder of abnormal platelet adhesion associated with low factor VIII activity. The von Willebrand factor is a large multimeric molecule which is encoded by a gene on chromosome 12. It is stored in Weibel–Palade bodies in endothelial cells and platelet α-granules. This protein is involved in platelet adhesion and is the carrier molecule for factor VIII, preventing its premature destruction. Inheritance is autosomal dominant and point mutations and major deletions of the gene have been described. Patients complain of post-traumatic bleeding and mucous membrane bleeding (eg epistaxis and menorrhagia). Laboratory features include prolonged bleeding time, reduced factor VIII levels, low von Willebrand factor levels and defective platelet aggregation with ristocetin. Treatment includes DDAVP which may boost factor VIII levels, factor VIII concentrates and fibrinolytic inhibitors (eg tranexamic acid).

2.45   B: Disseminated intravascular coagulation

In disseminated intravascular coagulation intravascular deposition of fibrin and consumption of coagulation factors and platelets result from release of procoagulant material or widespread endothelial damage. Microvascular thrombosis and bleeding is a consequence. The triggers include infections (eg *Clostridium welchii* septicaemia), malignancy (eg acute promyelocytic leukaemia), obstetric complications (amniotic fluid embolus, abruptio placenta, eclampsia and retained placenta), incompatible blood transfusion, widespread tissue damage, liver failure, severe burns, snake bites and vascular malformations. Laboratory tests may show haemolytic anaemia with red cell fragmentation on the blood film and major derangement of the coagulation screen with high levels of FDPs. It is most important to treat or remove the underlying cause and to support the patient with blood platelets, fresh frozen plasma and cryoprecipitate as indicated by the amount of derangement of the coagulation screen and the patient's clinical condition.

2.46   A: Acute lymphoblastic leukaemia

Acute lymphoblastic leukaemia is the common form of leukaemia in children with a peak incidence at three to four years. Clinical features include those due to bone marrow failure (anaemia, fever and infections, bruising and bleeding) and due to organ infiltration (tender bones, lymphadenopathy, splenomegaly and hepatomegaly, meningeal involvement, mediastinal compression and testicular swelling). The bone marrow is hypercellular with marked proliferation of blasts which are fully characterised using cytochemical and immunological markers. Management is initially supportive to correct for the consequences of bone marrow failure. Combinations of chemotherapy, including vincristine, daunorubicin, prednisolone and asparaginase are used to induce remission and further courses of treatment are administered to consolidate the remission. Treatment must be given to the central nervous system (methotrexate and radiotherapy) to prevent the appearance of disease there. Maintenance therapy is usually continued for two years. Prognosis in children is relatively good with over 90% achieving a remission and 70% remaining in first remission five years from diagnosis.

2.47   B: Hodgkin's disease

Hodgkin's disease is a malignant tumour arising in lymphoid tissue in which Reed–Sternberg and lymphocytic and histiocytic cells are described. Clinically, patients present with painless non-tender superficial lymphadenopathy. Cervical, axillary and inguinal nodes are commonly involved. Mediastinal involvement presenting as superior vena caval obstruction or pleural effusions is the presenting feature in approximately 10% of cases, frequently young women with the nodular sclerosing subtype. Splenomegaly occurs in 50% of cases at some point in the disease and cutaneous involvement is a late complication in 10%. Other organs, including bone, lung, gastrointestinal tract or brain are rarely involved. Constitutional symptoms include fever (Pel–Ebstein), pruritus, night sweats, weight loss, and alcohol-induced pain in affected nodes.

2.48   D: Primary thrombocythaemia

Primary thrombocythaemia is a disorder where there is megakaryocyte proliferation and overproduction of platelets. It is usually accepted that the platelet count should be greater than 600×10^9/l and another cause of a raised platelet count excluded. Causes which must be excluded include polycythaemia vera, chronic myeloid leukaemia and myelofibrosis and myelodysplasia, and reaction to haemorrhage, iron deficiency, malignancy, infection or post-splenectomy. The raised platelet count in primary thrombocythaemia can result in bleeding or thrombosis. Treatment involves the use of antiplatelet agents such as aspirin and lowering of the platelet count with hydroxyurea, anagrelide, interferon, busulfan or radioactive phosphorus.

2.49   C: Oral iron supplements

Meat, particularly liver, is a better source of iron than vegetables or dairy products. The average Western diet contains 10–15mg of iron daily of which only 10–15% is absorbed. Iron deficiency is manifest by a microcytic hypochromic anaemia with anisocytosis, pencil-shaped poikilocytes and target cells on the blood film. The cause of the iron deficiency must be treated, but the deficiency is best managed with oral iron. Ferrous sulphate 200 mg three times a day is the cheapest preparation and other preparations should only be used if this one cannot be tolerated. Optimal absorption is before food but this is often the worst tolerated way to take the preparation. The haemoglobin will rise at maximal rate of 1 g/dl per week and should be accompanied by a reticulocyte response. Parenteral iron can be given by intramuscular or intravenous routes but is only indicated if oral iron cannot be tolerated. The haemoglobin will not rise any faster if iron is administered by this route. Transfusion is not an effective way of replacing iron. It exposes the patient to the risks of transfusion and should only be used to correct life-threatening anaemia.

2.50   C: Methaemoglobinaemia induced by dapsone

Methaemoglobin is formed by the oxidation of haem iron from the ferrous to the ferric state. Methaemoglobinaemia results when the rate of formation of methaemoglobin exceeds its rate of removal by the normal cellular mechanisms which are NADH, NADPH and the methaemoglobin reductases. This can be caused by oxidising drugs which are capable of converting haemoglobin to methaemoglobin, for example dapsone, primaquine or lidocaine (lignocaine). It may also be due to a congenital defect due to a deficiency of NADH-cytochrome b5 reductase or the presence of an abnormal haemoglobin. Methaemoglobin is read at wavelengths similar to reduced haemoglobin and may cause falsely low readings with pulse oximetry.

2.51   D: Polycythaemia vera (PV)

The diagnostic criteria for polycythaemia vera are as follows:

A1 Raised red cell mass (> 25% above normal)
A2 Absence of a cause of secondary polycythaemia
A3 Palpable splenomegaly
A4 Acquired cytogenetic abnormality

B1 Thrombocytosis (platelets > 400 x 10^9/l)
B2 Neutrophil leukocytosis (neutrophil count > 10 x 10^9/l)
B3 Splenomegaly demonstrated on isotope/ultrasound scanning
B4 Characteristic BFU-E growth or reduced serum erythropoietin

A1 + A2 + A3 or A4 establishes PV. A1 + A2 + two of B establishes PV

2.52   B: Chronic lymphocytic leukaemia

Chronic lymphocytic leukaemia is characterised by a monoclonal population of lymphocytes in the blood and bone marrow. It represents 25% of all leukaemias and occurs in older patients with a male predominance. Clinically there may be painless lymphadenopathy and features of bone marrow replacement. Hepatosplenomegaly occurs with more advanced disease. Infections are common in the later stages due to neutropenia and immune deficiency. Lymphocytosis is seen with smear cells reported on the blood film. Patients with early-stage disease do not need treatment and may not progress for many years. Bone marrow failure should initially be treated with prednisolone. Alkalating agents can control the disease for long periods of time. The anti-purine agent fludarabine alone or in combination with cyclophosphamide is useful for second-line therapy and the monoclonal antibody CAMPATH is a new agent which may be effective in some cases.

2.53   C: Immune thrombocytopenic purpura

Immune thrombocytopenic purpura is a relatively common disorder, with its highest incidence in young women. Autoantibodies, frequently against the platelet glycoprotein IIa-IIIb complex, lead to removal of platelets from the circulation by the reticuloendothelial system and their destruction by macrophages in the spleen and throughout the reticuloendothelial system. In turn, platelet production can be increased up to five times normal. Clinically, patients present with easy bruising, petichial haemorrhage and menorrhagia. Mucosal bleeding can be a feature. Patients may recover spontaneously from an acute episode but steroids, splenectomy, high-dose intravenous immunoglobulin and immunosuppressive drugs such as azathioprine and cyclophosphamide may be required.

RESPIRATORY MEDICINE: 'BEST OF FIVE' ANSWERS

3.1   D: The alveoli have well-established collateral ventilation

The position of the heart and differing bronchial anatomy means that the right lung is usually larger than the left. The lingula is part of the left upper lobe. Terminal bronchioles lead into respiratory bronchioles, which in turn lead into alveolar ducts. Collateral ventilation takes place between alveoli via the pores of Kohn. There is active, neurally mediated widening of the glottic aperture during inspiration.

3.2   D: Nitrofurantion

Chemotherapeutic agents and immunosuppressants may result in diffuse lung disease which can closely resemble cryptogenic fibrosing alveolitis. Other drugs with similar effects include nitrofurantoin, amiodarone and hexamethonium (formerly used to treat hypertension). Ingestion of the weedkiller paraquat produces an acute and progressive, usually rapidly fatal, fibrosis.

3.3   E: Overall mortality is approximately 10%

Pneumocystis carinii pneumonia often presents with severe dyspnoea, dry cough, pyrexia and hypoxia. Chest X-ray may be normal in 10% but typically shows diffuse bilateral perihilar shadowing. Pleural effusion and lymphadenopathy is uncommon. Silver staining (not auramine) of the *Pneumocystis* organism (now classified as a fungus) is positive in over 90% of patients on lavage or induced sputum specimens. Arterial Po_2 and transfer factor are decreased. Treatment of choice is co-trimoxazole (co-triamterzide is a diuretic) but pentamidine may be given instead (intravenous or nebulised). Mortality following a first episode of *Pneumocystis carinii* pneumonia is less than 10% and secondary prophylaxis should be given (nebulised pentamidine, co-trimoxazole, dapsone or pyrimethamine). Tuberculosis and severe bacterial infection are commoner causes of opportunistic infection in HIV-positive Africans with AIDS. Mortality of PCP is about 10% (worse if ventilated).

3.4   E: The lower trachea is deviated to the right

In over 90% of normal subjects the right dome of the diaphragm is higher than the left; if much gas is present in the stomach they may temporarily be at the same level. Hilar shadows are composed of the pulmonary vessels and, to a small extent, the walls of the major bronchi. The centre of the right hilum is roughly opposite the third rib anteriorly; the left hilum is about 1 cm higher. Lingular pathology causes loss of clarity of the left heart border. The lower trachea is usually deviated to the right by the aorta.

3.5   B: Patients are still infectious once the rash has appeared

Chickenpox pneumonia is rare in children but may affect up to a third of adult cases. It is commoner in smokers. Patients continue to be infectious for a few days after the rash has appeared. Treatment is supportive as the majority of cases are self-limiting although aciclovir is used in severe cases (ventilation may also be necessary). Immunocompromised patients in contact with chickenpox may be given varicella immunoglobulin. Calcification on chest X-ray is well recognised. Other causes of calcification include healed tuberculosis, histoplasmosis and mitral stenosis. Secondary bacterial infection is commoner with measles virus and influenza pneumonia.

3.6   E: The total resistance in the pulmonary circulation is about 10% of that in the systemic circulation

Mean pulmonary artery pressure in a normal man is about 15 mmHg (2 kPa). The effects of gravity therefore mean that the apices of the lungs are barely perfused at all in the upright position. Resistance to pulmonary blood flow is about 10% of that in the systemic circulation. The carotid sinus is primarily a baroreceptor, the adjacent carotid body being the peripheral arterial chemoreceptor. Hypoxic stimulation of respiration occurs when PaO_2 is below about 65 mmHg (8.7kPa); usually, any tendency to a rise in $PaCO_2$ stimulates respiration before accompanying hypoxia does.

3.7   C: A decreased FEV_1/FVC is commonly seen in bronchiectasis

Total lung capacity is residual volume plus vital capacity. Spirometry measures tidal volume and inspiratory and expiratory reserve volumes which all add up to give the vital capacity. Residual volume (about 1.5 litres) and functional residual capacity (residual plus expiratory reserve volume) are not represented and need to be calculated indirectly. The peak flow measures maximal flow rate over 0.01 seconds and is a good predictor of large airway resistance. A reduced FEV_1/FVC ratio represents an obstructive picture and is seen in emphysema, chronic bronchitis and chronic severe asthma. In neuromuscular disease (respiratory muscle weakness) inspiratory and expiratory capacity decrease, TLC therefore falls and residual volume increases which decreases vital capacity. Note the FEV_1/VC ratio is normal. Spirometry rather than peak flow is used to monitor progression. Diaphragmatic weakness can be detected using lying and standing vital capacity. Standing vital capacity falls by 40–50% and patients may complain of breathlessness with immersion in water.

3.8   C: Ratio of residual volume/total lung capacity can be increased in COPD

Static lung volumes are total lung capacity (TLC), functional residual capacity (FRC) and residual volume (RV). They are measured by helium dilution (will miss bullae), which measures gas in communication with the airways, or body box plethysmography, which measures all intrathoracic (plus intra-abdominal) gas, including bullae and pneumothoraces. Volumes may be increased in asthma and emphysema due to air trapping. The RV/TLC ratio is increased when there is gas trapping, eg COPD. TLC is decreased with fibrosis.

3.9   B: Following treatment with oral itraconazole, *Aspergillus*-specific IgE decreases

Allergic bronchopulmonary aspergillosis is associated with thick sputum plugs and exacerbation of asthma in susceptible patients. Peripheral blood eosinophilia and raised serum IgE and specific IgE are characteristic. Chest X-ray/CT may show upper lobe infiltrates with proximal bronchiectasis. Precipitating antibodies (IgG) to *Aspergillus* antigen are weakly positive. Skin-prick testing often produces a rapid positive response. Treatment is with steroids and oral itraconazole. Intravenous amphotericin and flucytosine are used to treat invasive aspergillosis, which most commonly occurs in the immunosuppressed. Aspergilloma is treated conservatively or surgically if it is causing troublesome symptoms (haemoptysis).

3.10   B: Asthma

Carbon monoxide (CO) transfer factor measures gas transfer between alveoli and blood. Usually, a single breath of gas containing a known low concentration of CO is taken, held for 10 seconds, then expired. Measurement of expired gas volume and CO concentration enables calculation of CO uptake by blood flowing through pulmonary capillaries. When free blood is present in the bronchial tree, transfer factor is high as the haemoglobin binds the CO (also high in polycythaemia). Gas transfer is normal/high in asthmatics, but reduced in patients with emphysema due to destruction of gas exchanging surface and mismatching of ventilation and perfusion. A normal transfer factor in a bronchitic or emphysematous patient should always raise the possibility of asthma.

3.11 E: Isoniazid is predominantly bactericidal in action

Pyridoxine is given to prevent isoniazid neuropathy. Apart from thiacetazone and PAS (para-aminosalicylic acid), most of the antituberculous drugs are bactericidal, with isoniazid the most potent. Ethambutol is bacteriostatic and can cause optic (retrobulbar) neuritis as a side-effect, resulting in reduced visual acuity, central scotoma and disturbance of red-green perception. Rifampicin induces liver enzymes, thus reducing the half-life of warfarin, the oral contraceptive pill and phenytoin. It is excreted into the bile duct and is safe in renal failure. Rifampicin accelerates the metabolism of corticosteroids and in Addison's disease cortisol must be increased in dose by 50%. Other well-recognised side-effects of rifampicin include rash, abnormal liver function, hepatitis and thrombocytopenia.

3.12 C: Flow/volume loop

PEFR and the FEV_1 to FVC ratio will be low in both asthma and upper airways obstruction. The two tests together may be useful, since in upper airways obstruction PEFR is usually (but not always) disproportionately reduced compared with FEV_1. The FEV_1 (ml) divided by PEFR (l/min) is usually less than 10. Values greater than 10 are very suggestive of large airways obstruction. Inspection of typical flow/volume loops, the best physiological test for distinguishing asthma from upper airways obstruction, will help explain why this is the case.

3.13 A: Extrinsic allergic alveolitis

Extrinsic allergic alveolitis, largely due to type III and IV hypersensitivity (immune complex and cell-mediated), is characteristically not associated with eosinophilia. *Ascaris lumbricoides*, *Ancylostoma braziliense* and *Trichuris trichiura* are the commonest parasites associated with pulmonary shadows and eosinophilia. Aspirin, para-aminosalicylic acid, phenylbutazone, nitrofurantoin and methotrexate may also be responsible. *Aspergillus fumigatus* is the commonest cause of so-called asthmatic pulmonary eosinophilia in Great Britain. Lung involvement and eosinophilia are present in about a third of cases of polyarteritis nodosa.

3.14   C: Arterial P_{O_2} is normal or high

The high hydrogen ion concentration in a metabolic acidosis stimulates the respiratory centre and hyperventilation occurs; arterial P_{O_2} thus tends to be high and P_{CO_2} is low. Bicarbonate buffer is used up and plasma bicarbonate falls; the carbonic acid generated by this process is itself buffered initially by haemoglobin and subsequently leads to increased CO_2 output by the lungs. Acidosis shifts the oxygen dissociation curve of haemoglobin to the right (ie affinity falls). At tissue P_{O_2} the haemoglobin can carry less oxygen than formerly and more is given up to the tissues. Acidosis shifts potassium from intracellular to extracellular compartments. Urinary excretion of potassium increases, so patients may be whole-body potassium-depleted despite having high plasma potassium levels.

3.15   C: Myasthenia gravis

Cor pulmonale is caused by hypoxaemic respiratory failure (P_{O_2} less than 60 mmHg/8 kPa) which leads to pulmonary hypertension, leading to right-sided cardiac failure. ECG may show right axis deviation, right bundle branch block and right ventricular hypertrophy. Chest X-ray may show enlarged pulmonary arteries and evidence of lung disease. Patients with cor pulmonale have a poor prognosis. Approximately two-thirds are dead within five years. Pulmonary hypertension may be reduced with long-term oxygen therapy, and diuretics will relieve peripheral oedema. In mitral stenosis raised left atrial pressure, and not hypoxia, leads to pulmonary hypertension and right-sided cardiac failure.

3.16   B: Emphysematous changes in the lower lobes suggest α_1-antitrypsin deficiency

Compliance measures stretchability (volume change per unit pressure). Its reciprocal is elastance (elastic recoil). Compliance is increased in emphysema and falls with pulmonary fibrosis. Emphysema due to α_1-antitrypsin deficiency affects the lower lobes predominantly. Homozygotes for the deficiency gene have low levels of α_1-antitrypsin (ZZ = levels 10% normal, MZ = levels 60% normal). Clinical features are worse in smokers and there may be associated cirrhosis. Neonatal jaundice is a rare childhood presentation. Cardiac arrhythmias, notably multifocal ventricular ectopics, are seen with both emphysema and chronic bronchitis (many patients in practice have both), particularly in the presence of hypoxia and pulmonary hypertension. The anatomic dead space which acts to filter, warm and humidify air comprises the mouth, nasopharynx, trachea and bronchi (150 ml). The functional dead space is the same plus any alveolar volume where there is no gas exchange.

3.17   A: Occupational asbestos exposure

Asbestos is the correct answer because of the bilateral calcification. Very extensive pleural calcification is likely to be due to old tuberculosis or haemothorax. Calcified pleural plaques may be difficult to see radiologically *en face*, but may be more readily visible along the lateral chest wall or on the diaphragmatic pleura. Oblique radiographs may help. Pleural calcification is not a feature of coal-worker's pneumoconiosis or chickenpox pneumonia: the latter may result in miliary calcification of the lung fields. Other rare causes of pleural calcification include chronic pancreatitis, chronic haemodialysis, calcified metastases, and alveolar microlithiasis.

3.18   E: Tuberculous meningitis co-exists in about a third of patients

Miliary tuberculosis results from haematogenous dissemination of tubercle bacilli. The classic radiographic picture of multiple millet seed-size (1–2 mm) pulmonary lesions gives the condition its name but the chest X-ray may be normal for months before development of miliary shadows. Patients, particularly the elderly, may be mildly unwell with only unexplained anaemia or fever for long periods before diagnosis. The tuberculin test may be negative, particularly in the very ill. Hypokalaemia is well recognised but poorly understood. Approximately 30% of adults with miliary tuberculosis have tuberculous meningitis at the time of presentation.

3.19   E: Arterial blood Po_2 (95 mmHg/12.4 kPa) is less than alveolar Po_2 because of arterio-venous shunting

Haemoglobin has four haem subunits, each of which combines with one molecule of oxygen. Affinity for oxygen is enhanced after binding of the first molecule, which increases further with the second molecule and so on. This explains the sigmoid shape of the oxygen saturation curve. A shift to the left increases the slope because affinity of haemoglobin for oxygen has been increased. Decreased temperature, 2,3 DPG, CO_2 and a rise in pH all shift the curve to the left. A shift to the right means decreased affinity of haemoglobin for oxygen and is caused by increases in temperature, 2,3 DPG, CO_2 and a fall in pH. At tissue level Pco_2 rises and pH falls and the affinity of haemoglobin for oxygen falls, allowing oxygen to dissociate. This is the Bohr effect and the reverse happens in the lungs. Myoglobin and fetal haemoglobin bind oxygen more readily and shift the curve to the left.

3.20   A: Smoking increases the clearance of theophylline

Theophylline is a methylxanthine similar to caffeine (strong coffee has a bronchodilator effect). Increased clearance occurs with smoking, enzyme induction (rifampicin, alcohol), childhood, and with barbecued meat. Levels are increased by ciprofloxacin and erythromycin, cardiac failure and liver disease. Beta-agonists are more effective bronchodilators than anticholinergics. Ipratropium can cause prostatic hypertrophy. In acute asthma high levels of circulating catecholamines, β-agonists and steroids can lead to hypokalaemia. Steroids inhibit interleukin and granulocyte-macrophage colony-stimulating factor, thus reducing the inflammatory response. Inhaled steroids do not cause growth suppression in children and there may be a growth spurt as asthma is controlled.

3.21   D: Adenosine via pulmonary artery catheter may be used as an acute vasodilator

Primary pulmonary hypertension affects young adults, women more than men. It is diagnosed if the mean pulmonary artery pressure is greater than 25 mmHg at rest or 30 mmHg on exercise in the presence of a cardiac output less than 5 l/min. Secondary causes include chronic obstructive pulmonary disease, chronic thromboembolism, pulmonary fibrosis and thoracic deformity. Clinical features include a loud second heart sound, cyanosis, right ventricular heave, prominent *a* wave in the JVP, third and fourth heart sounds. There may be tricuspid and pulmonary regurgitation and peripheral oedema. In primary disease acute vasodilator therapy is with prostacyclin or adenosine; the chronic therapy most frequently used is calcium-channel blockers (nifedipine, diltiazem), with ACE inhibitors being less effective. Prognosis is poor and many patients are now referred for heart-lung transplantation.

3.22   C: Daytime insomnolence

The systemic hypertension often seen in patients with obstructive sleep apnoea is poorly understood. Pulmonary hypertension and secondary polycythaemia are thought to result from the hypoxaemia that accompanies the episodes of apnoea, and which in some individuals may persist during waking hours. Daytime somnolence is characteristic; patients may fall asleep whilst driving, eating or talking. Depression affects at least 25% of patients.

3.23 D: Hypertrophic pulmonary osteoarthropathy can resolve if the primary tumour is treated

Small-cell carcinoma has a short doubling time of 30 days and has usually spread by the time of presentation. Combination chemotherapy with agents such as cyclophosphamide, vincristine, etoposide, adriamycin and methotrexate have been tried. Studies have suggested that six cycles of treatment at three- to four-week intervals is optimal. No survival advantage was noted in having further courses or maintenance chemotherapy. Adriamycin is cardiotoxic. Vincristine causes demyelination leading to peripheral neuropathy. Most cytotoxic agents are myelotoxic. Cisplatin is nephrotoxic and can also cause a sensory peripheral neuropathy and tinnitus. HPOA is rare in small-cell lung carcinoma and commonest in squamous cell carcinoma. It is associated with finger clubbing in 90% of cases and may also improve with vagotomy.

3.24 B: Eaton–Lambert syndrome occurs most commonly with small cell carcinoma

Ectopic ACTH causes a hypokalaemic metabolic alkalosis. Some patients develop pigmentation due to melanocyte-stimulating hormone production. It occurs with small cell lung carcinoma (SCLC) where the natural history is too short for features of Cushing's syndrome to develop. Progressive proximal muscle weakness, dysphagia and dry mouth are characteristic of Eaton–Lambert syndrome. EMG reveals post-tetanic potentiation and muscles get stronger with repeat contraction. SIADH reveals a dilutional hyponatraemia, low plasma osmolality (less than 260 mosmol/kg) and a high urine osmolality. Treatment is with demeclocycline which causes a nephrogenic diabetes insipidus by competing for ADH at the renal tubule. In this context SIADH is almost always associated with SLC and will improve following chemotherapy. The commonest cause of hypercalcaemia is bony metastases, though squamous cell tumours occasionally exhibit ectopic PTH secretion.

3.25 A: Bronchiectasis

Acute lung abscess would not cause clubbing. BAC patients tend to produce copious amounts of non-purulent sputum. Fibrosing alveolitis tends to cause fine crackles and a dry cough. Sarcoidosis patients do not show clubbing.

3.26   D: Lymphangioleiomyomatosis

Lymphangioleiomyomatosis is confined to women of childbearing age and presents most commonly as a spontaneous pneumothorax on the background of previously undiagnosed cystic lung disease. There is evidence of marked smooth muscle hypertrophy, which appears to be at least partially oestrogen-driven. Oophorectomy, progesterone treatment and lung transplantation are all options. Langerhans' cell histiocytosis occurs predominantly in cigarette smokers but sarcoidosis and extrinsic allergic alveolitis are relatively uncommon in smoking. This latter effect is believed to be the result of cigarette smoking impairing MHC class II expression on alveolar macrophages, and thus antigen presentation to CD4 T lymphocytes (helper T cells).

3.27   E: Sputum cytology

Both the speed and method of diagnosis of lung cancer are very emotive and one of the most important points to take into account is the general state of the patient. Hence this elderly patient with poor lung function and low Po_2 is clearly not fit for invasive investigations, let alone radical treatment (so here sputum cytology is worth remembering). In fact, when three to four sputum samples are collected from patients there is a diagnostic rate of around 70–80%. With an FEV_1 of only 0.8 litres, she is likely to be poorly tolerant of a pneumothorax, which may result from a percutaneous biopsy.

3.28   D: Pleural aspiration alone

In a patient with a small pneumothorax and otherwise normal lungs, it is likely to take three to six weeks for the pneumothorax to resolve without intervention. The rate of resorption for a pneumothorax, once the leak has sealed, is 1.25% of hemithorax volume per day. A complete pneumothorax should not be left untreated as pleural adhesions may develop, making subsequent re-expansion more difficult. A patient with chronic lung disease must be admitted, as the risk of respiratory compromise is greater. Indications for aspiration include any significant dyspnoea or complete collapse. Aspiration should be stopped if there is resistance, excessive coughing, or 2.5 litres of gas have been aspirated. The indications for intercostal tube drainage are (a) failed simple aspiration, (b) tension pneumothorax, (c) significant bleeding into the pleural space. For pure pneumothoraces, a 20-Fr chest tube should suffice but a size 28+ should be used for haemothorax or empyema.

3.29   A: Echocardiography

This patient is at one extreme of pulmonary embolism presentation. Those with a massive life-threatening episode, caused by a central embolism, present shocked and extremely unwell (as in this case). These patients need rapid diagnosis, exclusion of other possible causes of such a presentation, such as aortic dissection, MI, cardiac tamponade and rapid thrombolysis. The most time- and cost-effective method of diagnosing such a large central PE is by echocardiography. This is the current recommendation from the BTS working group. Another method is by spiral CT but not all hospitals have this form of imaging available as yet.

3.30   A: Cryptogenic organising pneumonia

Transient X-ray shadowing narrows the large list of diffuse parenchymal lung diseases right down to a much more manageable number. Such a presentation can occur in Churg–Strauss, EAA, eosinophilic pneumonia, pulmonary haemorrhage, allergic bronchopulmonary aspergillosis (ABPA) and COP, though only Churg–Strauss is associated with a positive ANCA.

3.31   A: Gram-negative *Enterobacteriaceae*

Streptococcus pneumoniae causes 39% of hospitalised CAP, *Mycoplasma pneumoniae* 10.8%, *Legionella* 3.6%, *S. aureus* 1.9%, Gram-negative *Enterobacteriaceae* 1.0%. For CAP severe enough to necessitate ICU, the figures are 21.6%, 2.7%, 17.8%, 8.7% and 1.6% respectively. So, although *Legionella* and *S. aureus* are uncommon causes of CAP, they become more important when looking at severe CAP (BTS Guidelines on CAP, December 2001).

3.32   C: *Streptococcus pneumoniae* is an unlikely pathogen in pneumonia associated with HIV infection

With the exception of 'C' the statements are all true. In HIV infection, when the CD4 count is still reasonably preserved, pulmonary infection with bacteria and tuberculosis are common. The commonest aetiology for pneumonia remains *Streptococcus pneumoniae* in this group.

3.33   E: Urinary antigen testing

Legionella pneumonia is usually caused by *Legionella pneumophila* serotype 1. Gram stain would not identify *Legionella* and culture, if performed for this pathogen, would be delayed. Serology may be unreliable and will usually require both an acute and convalescent sample (weeks apart) allowing a retrospective diagnosis. Urinary antigen testing specific for serotype 1 only is a rapid test commercially available. Soluble antigen is excreted in the urine for one to three weeks during the acute pneumonia.

3.34   E: Total pulmonary compliance is increased

The shape of the thorax changes in pregnancy because (a) the AP and transverse diameters of the thorax increase by ~ 2 cm and (b) the diaphragm gradually gets pushed upwards by the increasing size of the gravid uterus, to a maximum of 4 cm. These two effects combine to decrease the chest wall (and therefore total pulmonary) compliance, which causes an increase in breathing during pregnancy. As tidal volume increases, this increases minute ventilation, which is the product of V_T x RR (respiratory rate). As alveolar ventilation and $Paco_2$ are inversely related, an increase in the former will result in a decrease in the latter. Therefore, a mild respiratory alkalosis develops, which is compensated for by increased bicarbonate excretion by the kidneys to maintain normal pH.

3.35   E: 15% of normal

The normal genotype is MM homozygote (100% levels) and occurs in 86% of the UK population. Following this (with levels in brackets) are MS (75%), MZ (57%), SS (52%), SZ (37%) and ZZ (16%).

3.36   A: 0.5 ml adrenaline 1:1000 intramuscularly

Life-saving treatment for acute anaphylaxis is adrenaline, administered as 0.5 ml (for adults), 1:1000 intramuscularly. The intravenous 1:10, 000 preparation can cause severe arrhythmia such as ventricular tachycardia, and is therefore only appropriate in the event of immediately life-threatening cardiogenic shock or cardiac arrest. Intravenous antihistamines and hydrocortisone are also useful therapies in acute anaphylaxis, but their administration is secondary in importance to life-saving treatment with adrenaline.

3.37   D: 0.1 ml of 1:1000 intradermally

A standard Mantoux test requires the insertion of 10 tuberculin units (TU) intradermally. The test is read at 48–72 hours and the transverse diameter of induration (ie how much is palpable), not erythema, is measured and recorded. Confusion arises because of the way the Mantoux concentration is recorded.

    1:100   = 1000   TU/ml (100 TU/0.1 ml)
    1:1000   = 100   TU/ml (10 TU/0.1 ml)
    1:10, 000 = 10   TU/ml (1 TU/0.1 ml)

3.38   E: VA 100   Kco 50

Churg–Strauss, being a small vessel vasculitis, will primarily affect the pulmonary vascular bed (but have no effect on the effective ventilatory volume of the lung). Thus, only the Kco will be affected and the VA will remain normal, though together giving the combination of a Tlco of 50% predicted.

3.39   A: Bi-level positive airway pressure (BiPAP)

This question highlights the problem of how to manage a patient with hypercapnic hypoxaemic respiratory failure. The patient cannot be left with that degree of hypoxaemia owing to the sigmoid shape of the Hb-O_2 dissociation curve. The initial PaO_2 of 5.3 kPa represents a haemoglobin oxygen saturation of ~70–75%. It is SaO_2, rather than PaO_2 that ultimately determines O_2 delivery to the tissues. Clearly the inspired oxygen concentration required increasing but this has resulted in the $PaCO_2$ to rising sufficiently high to render the patient acidotic. Whilst intubation may be appropriate in some cases of COPD, it is less likely to be appropriate in the absence of a clearly identifiable reversible pulmonary insult. Non-invasive ventilation is a more appropriate management step and in this case, with severe COPD, BiPAP is preferable to CPAP because of the ability to set a lower expiratory positive pressure and allow the patient with obstructive lung disease to breathe out against the positive pressure.

3.40   B: Bronchoalveolar lavage lymphocytosis

BAL lymphocytosis predicts a better corticosteroid response than the more usual BAL neutrophilia, which is associated with a worse corticosteroid response. A $PaO_2 > 8.0$ kPa (60 mmHg) on air, tells us that the patient is teetering on respiratory failure. Pulmonary hypertension and right ventricular failure may develop with more severe hypoxaemia (cor pulmonale). Predominant reticular pattern on HRCT correlates with predominant fibrosis (irreversible) rather than the ground-glass appearance that can correlate with a more inflammatory (potentially reversible) pattern of disease. However, ground-glass is simply a CT pattern that arises from displacement of air, which can occur because of inflammation, fluid, fine fibrosis and during normal expiration. Rapid DTPA clearance is abnormal and may identify a subgroup who may develop progressive disease. However, DTPA is of more predictive value when it is normal/slow (normal > 40 minutes), when it tends to predict stability over the ensuing one to three years.

3.41   C: Asbestosis

The elevated forced expiratory ratio (FEV_1/FVC) confirms a restrictive ventilatory defect. The low lung volumes cause the T_{LCO} to drop. However, if this was due to pure extrathoracic restriction (mesothelioma, diffuse pleural thickening) then one would expect the transfer coefficient (K_{CO}) to be normal/supranormal because all the cardiac output is going through essentially normal but smaller-volume lungs. Asbestos plaques are a 'signature' of asbestos exposure and are not usually problematic *per se*. Asbestosis is interstitial lung disease secondary to asbestos and would cause all the lung function abnormalities described. Asbestosis does not respond to corticosteroids and the best advice is to avoid further exposure and to encourage smoking cessation. The risk of bronchial carcinoma is over 50 times higher in a smoker with asbestos exposure compared to someone with neither exposure.

3.42   E: 24-hour urinary calcium of 12 mmol/l

The indications for using corticosteroids include hypercalcaemia/hypercalciuria, rapidly worsening pulmonary function tests, ocular involvement, cardiac involvement, CNS involvement, lupus pernio. Normal 24-hour urinary calcium is 2.5–7.5 mmol/l.

3.43   A: CT thorax with 2-mm slices

This question requires the knowledge that high-resolution CT (HRCT) uses thin sections, ie 2 mm. When looking at interstitial lung diseases, HRCT is used because of the higher quality detail of the images. One caveat of HRCT is that slices may be taken 10–20 mm apart and can potentially miss small masses. This can be overcome by performing contiguous thick sections (10 mm) at the same time. MRI of the thorax is more useful when looking at mediastinal structures rather than fine parenchymal disease. PET scanning can be used to assess pulmonary inflammation but in clinical practice is mainly restricted to lung cancer. DTPA assesses alveolar permeability and can help when trying to predict whether a patient's disease will progress or be stable. DTPA is affected by cigarette smoking and should not be performed for at least four weeks after smoking cessation.

3.44   A: Fibrosing alveolitis

Pulmonary vascular disease with pulmonary hypertension tends to occur more frequently in those with the anticentromere autoantibody. Fibrosing alveolitis is more likely with the Scl-70 autoantibody. Organising pneumonia tends to occur with polymyositis/dermatomyositis and rheumatoid disease. Shrinking lung occurs in SLE and is thought to occur because of diaphragmatic myopathy. Aspiration pneumonia can occur in systemic sclerosis because of oesophageal dysmotility.

3.45   D: Ipsilateral supraclavicular lymph node metastasis

Lung cancer is inoperable if: stage IIIB or worse; pleural effusion (if malignant aetiology); nerve entrapment (phrenic or recurrent laryngeal); SVC obstruction; distant metastases; FEV_1 less than 1.0–1.5 litres. As far as TNM staging is concerned, any N3 (contralateral hilar or mediastinal nodes) or any T4 (any tumour of any size with invasion of mediastinum or involving heart, great vessels, trachea, oesophagus, vertebral body, carina, or malignant pleural effusion) tumour is considered inoperable.

3.46   C: FEV$_1$ less than 1.5 litres

LTOT for COPD should be prescribed for those with a PaO_2 < 7.3 kPa (55 mmHg), with or without hypercapnia, and an FEV$_1$ < 1.5 litres. LTOT should be considered in those with PaO_2 between 7.3 and 8.0 kPa, and pulmonary hypertension, nocturnal oxygen desaturation or peripheral oedema. Blood gas tensions should be checked when the patient is stable on maximal treatment, on at least two occasions three weeks apart. LTOT needs to be given for at least 15 hours per day to achieve benefit (five-year survival increase from 25% to 41%).

3.47   E: Malignant pleural effusion

Very high pleural fluid eosinophil counts suggest intrapleural blood or air. Other causes of pleural fluid eosinophilia include drug reactions, asbestos-related effusions, fungal and parasitic pleural infections. Pleural fluid eosinophilia makes tuberculosis and malignancy less likely.

3.48   D: Leiomyoma of the oesophagus

Anterior mediastinal masses include thymus, thyroid, parathyroid, germ cell tumours and Morgagni's hernia. Posterior mediastinal masses tend to be either oesophageal, neural, vascular or Bochdalek's hernia. Middle mediastinal masses are either pericardial, vascular or cardiac. All the above assume the mass is confined to a single compartment only.

3.49   C: Increase in lung elastic recoil

The four 1994 American-European criteria for diagnosing ARDS are: acute onset; PaO_2 / FiO_2 ratio $\leq$ 200 mmHg (irrespective of PEEP level); bilateral infiltrates on chest X-ray; pulmonary capillary wedge pressure $\leq$ 18 mmHg. Pulmonary compliance is decreased in ARDS (ie stiff lungs) and therefore elastic recoil is increased.

3.50   D: Multidrug-resistant TB (MDRTB) requires the addition of two or more drugs at a time in a failing regimen

Multidrug-resistant TB (MDRTB) requires the addition of two or more drugs at a time in a failing regimen; otherwise the organism may become successively resistant to all agents. Some patients with sputum smear-positive TB may be managed at home provided that they avoid contact with non-exposed individuals for at least two weeks (by which time they should be non-infectious if compliant with appropriate therapy). Rifampicin and isoniazid may be used if the patient is HIV-positive. Corticosteroids are sometimes used in patients with refractory constitutional symptoms, eg fever. Ethambutol may cause retrobulbar neuropathy, and so patients should be warned about loss of visual acuity and red-green discrimination, and should discontinue treatment and seek advice if this occurs.

REVISION CHECKLISTS

CARDIOLOGY: REVISION CHECKLIST

Valvular heart disease

- ☐ Heart sounds
- ☐ Mitral stenosis
- ☐ Valve lesions/murmurs
- ☐ Antibiotic prophylaxis
- ☐ Catheterisation data
- ☐ Mitral valve prolapse

Arrhythmias

- ☐ Wolff–Parkinson–White/SVT
- ☐ Atrial fibrillation
- ☐ Ventricular tachycardia
- ☐ LBBB
- ☐ Prolonged Q T interval
- ☐ Torsades de pointes

Pericardial and myocardial disease

- ☐ Constrictive pericarditis
- ☐ Cardiac tamponade
- ☐ Pericardial effusion
- ☐ IHD/heart muscle disease
- ☐ Myocardial infarction
- ☐ Cardiomyopathy
- ☐ Left ventricular failure
- ☐ Unstable angina
- ☐ Coronary bypass surgery
- ☐ Left ventricular hypertrophy
- ☐ Signs underlying heart disease

Congenital heart disease

- ☐ Cyanotic heart disease/ Eisenmenger's
- ☐ ASD
- ☐ Patent ductus arteriosus
- ☐ VSD

Large vessel disease

- ☐ Pulmonary embolus
- ☐ Aortic dissection
- ☐ Pulmonary hypertension

Miscellaneous

- ☐ Cannon *a* waves in JVP
- ☐ Alcohol and the heart
- ☐ Carotid body/cardiac sympathetics
- ☐ Coronary circulation
- ☐ Left atrial myxoma

HAEMATOLOGY: REVISION CHECKLIST

Red cell physiology and anaemias

- ☐ Iron deficiency/metabolism/therapy
- ☐ Macrocytosis/pernicious anaemia
- ☐ Folate deficiency
- ☐ Basophilia
- ☐ Erythropoiesis/haemoglobin physiology
- ☐ Haem biosynthesis
- ☐ Sideroblastic anaemia
- ☐ Aplastic anaemia
- ☐ Investigation of anaemia
- ☐ Vitamin B_{12} metabolism

Haemolytic anaemia

- ☐ Haemolytic anaemia
- ☐ Sickle cell/haemoglobinopathy
- ☐ Hereditary spherocytosis
- ☐ Reticulocytosis
- ☐ G6PD deficiency
- ☐ Haemolytic-uraemic syndrome
- ☐ Intravascular haemolysis

Bleeding disorders

- ☐ Thrombocytopenia
- ☐ Haemophilia
- ☐ Bleeding time
- ☐ Fresh frozen plasma
- ☐ von Willebrand's disease

Haematological malignancy

- ☐ Hodgkin's/non-Hodgkin's lymphoma
- ☐ Leukaemia
- ☐ Pancytopenia/splenomegaly
- ☐ Polycythaemia

Miscellaneous

- ☐ Hyposplenism
- ☐ Methaemoglobinaemia
- ☐ Neutropenia
- ☐ Thrombocytosis
- ☐ Bone infarction
- ☐ Bone marrow test
- ☐ Eosinophilia
- ☐ Hyperuricaemia and haematological disease
- ☐ Paroxysmal nocturnal haemoglobinuria

RESPIRATORY MEDICINE: REVISION CHECKLIST

Respiratory infections

- ☐ Pneumonia
- ☐ Bronchopulmonary aspergillosis
- ☐ Acute bronchiolitis
- ☐ Psittacosis
- ☐ Viral infections
- ☐ TB

Lung cancer

- ☐ Bronchial carcinoma
- ☐ Surgery for cancer
- ☐ Pancoast's tumour
- ☐ Small-cell cancer
- ☐ Mesothelioma

Pulmonary physiology

- ☐ Lung function tests
- ☐ Normal physiology
- ☐ Transfer factor
- ☐ Forced hyperventilation

End-stage lung disease

- ☐ Respiratory failure
- ☐ Long-term oxygen

Interstitial lung disease/fibrosis

- ☐ Extrinsic allergic alveolitis
- ☐ Bronchiectasis
- ☐ ARDS
- ☐ Sarcoidosis
- ☐ Emphysema
- ☐ Fibrosing alveolitis
- ☐ Pulmonary fibrosis
- ☐ Asbestosis
- ☐ Cystic fibrosis

Miscellaneous

- ☐ Asthma
- ☐ Sleep-apnoea syndrome
- ☐ Autoimmune disease and the lung
- ☐ Abnormal chest X-ray
- ☐ Lung cavitation
- ☐ Pulmonary eosinophilia
- ☐ Pleural effusion

INDEX

Locators refer to question number.

Haematology

PASTEST BOOKS FOR MRCP PART 1

MRCP 1 Pocket Book Series
Further titles in this range:

Book 2:	Basic Sciences, Neurology, Psychiatry	*1 901198 80 4*
Book 3:	Endocrinology, Gastroenterology, Nephrology	*1 901198 85 5*
Book 4:	Clinical Pharmacology, Infectious Diseases, Immunology, Rheumatology	*1 901198 90 1*

Essential Revision Notes for MRCP: Revised Edition
Philip Kalra   *1 901198 59 6*
A definitive guide to revision for the MRCP examination that offers 19 chapters of informative material necessary to gain a successful exam result.

MRCP 1: Best of Five Practice Papers
Khalid Binymin   *1 901198 88 X*
Four practice papers with 100 questions in each. Excellent up-to-date clinical scenarios.

MRCP 1 'Best of Five' Multiple Choice Revision Book
Khalid Binymin   *1 901198 57 X*
This book features subject-based chapters ensuring all topics are fully covered.

MRCP 1 300 Best of Five
Geraint Rees   *1 901198 97 9*
300 brand new 'Best of Five' questions with excellent clinical scenarios encountered in everyday hospital practice.

MRCP 1: Best of Five Key Topic Summaries: Third Edition
Stephen Waring & Paul O'Neill   *1 904627 05 6*
Subject-based chapters in 'Best of Five' format with excellent clinical scenarios.

Essential Lists for MRCP
Stuart McPherson   *1 901198 58 8*
The lists contained in this book offer a compilation of clinical, diagnostic, investigative and prognostic features of the symptoms and diseases that cover the whole spectrum of general medicine. It is invaluable for MRCP Part 1 AND Part 2.

MRCP 1 Multiple True/False Revision Book
Philip Kalra   *1 901198 95 2*
600 multiple true/false questions in subject-based chapters and three 'test yourself' practice exams to give experience of exam fomat.

MCQs in Basic Medical Sciences for MRCP Part 1
Philippa Easterbrook   *1 906896 34 7*
300 exam-based MCQs focusing on basic sciences with expanded teaching notes.

PASTEST – DEDICATED TO YOUR SUCCESS

PasTest has been publishing books for doctors for over 30 years. Our extensive experience means that we are always one step ahead when it comes to knowledge of current trends and content of the Royal College exams.

We use only the best authors and lecturers, many of whom are Consultants and Royal College Examiners, which enables us to tailor our books and courses to meet your revision needs. We incorporate feedback from candidates to ensure that our books are continually improved.

This commitment to quality ensures that students who buy a PasTest book or attend a PasTest course achieve successful exam results.

Delivery to your Door

With a busy lifestyle, nobody enjoys walking to the shops for something that may or may not be in stock. Let us take away the hassle and deliver direct to your door. We will despatch your book within 24 hours of receiving your order. We also offer free delivery on books for medical students to UK addresses.

How to Order:

🖥 www.pastest.co.uk

To order books safely and securely online, shop at our website.

☎ Telephone: +44 (0)1565 752000

📠 Fax: +44 (0)1565 650264

✉ PasTest Ltd, FREEPOST, Knutsford, WA16 7BR.